Contents

Acknowledgments, ix

Introduction, 1

PART ONE

Deciding Whether
Back Surgery Is for You

1. Understanding Your Back, 7

2. Determining the Cause of
Your Back Problem, 19

3. Nonsurgical Treatment
Options, 37

4. Surgical Options, 55

PART TWO

Before and After
Your Back Surgery

5. Preparing for Surgery, 89

6. Your Successful Recovery, 111

PART THREE

A Healthy Back for Life

7. Preventing Future Back Problems, 131

8. Psychology and Back Pain, 149

Conclusion, 161

Selected References, 165

Resource List, 167

Index, 169

BACK SURGERY

Is It Right for You?

Edwin Haronian, MD

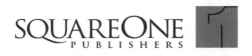

SQUAREONE
PUBLISHERS

The information and advice in this book are based on the training, personal experiences, and research of the author. Its contents are current and accurate; however, the information presented is not intended to substitute for professional medical advice. The author and the publisher urge you to consult with your physician or other qualified health-care provider prior to starting any treatment or undergoing any surgical procedure. Because there is always some risk involved, the author and publisher cannot be responsible for any adverse effects or consequences resulting from the use of any of the suggestions, preparations, or procedures described in this book.

COVER DESIGNER: Jeannie Tudor
TYPESETTER: Gary A. Rosenberg

Square One Publishers
115 Herricks Road
Garden City Park, NY 11040
(516) 535-2010 • (877) 900-BOOK
www.squareonepublishers.com

Library of Congress Cataloging-in-Publication Data

Haronian, Edwin.
  Back surgery : is it right for you? / Edwin Haronian.
    p. cm.
  ISBN-13: 978-0-7570-0276-2 (quality pbk.)
  ISBN-10: 0-7570-0276-5 (quality pbk.)
  1. Back--Surgery--Popular works. I. Title.

RD768.H367 2007
617.5'6059--dc22

                                         2007031473

Printed in the United States of America

10   9   8   7   6   5   4   3   2   1

To my newborn son,
who changed my life overnight;
and to my wife, who supported me
throughout this adventure.
I also dedicate this book to all the patients
who are struggling to make the right decision
about their health, and to all of my patients who
placed their trust in me to better their lives.

Acknowledgments

Many people helped create this book. However, I would especially like to acknowledge Lisa Messinger, whose work and guidance have been an invaluable source of motivation throughout. Her knowledge and experience ensured a writing style that is easy to read and understand. Special thanks to Dr. Ash Emrani, who sparked the writing of this book. Finally, I sincerely thank Dr. William Dillin, who taught me the art of spine surgery at the Kerlan-Jobe Orthopedic Clinic in Los Angeles.

BACK SURGERY: IS IT RIGHT FOR YOU?

Introduction

I wish I could say you are unique, but if you are holding this book, chances are you have joined one of the world's largest clubs. You have back pain—anything from a slight, nagging ache, to excruciating spasms that affect every aspect of your life. With these symptoms, you have become one of the four in five people who suffer from back pain at some point in their lives, making back-related disorders the most common of any medical ailment. You may possibly become one of the 500,000 people who have back surgery each year, or one of the additional million considering it.

Whether you are a business executive who first noticed distress while tapping the computer keys at your desk, a contractor who felt the pang while lugging heavy supplies to a job, or a young mother who can no longer lift her precious child, chances are it's more than just the pain that's distressing you. It's the often bewildering array of treatment options. In addition to a number of sophisticated surgeries from which to select, there are many nonsurgical options. As top sources such as *The New England Journal of Medicine* and the American Medical Association have commented recently, that leaves the confusing decision up to you.

I am thrilled to offer you a quick, convenient, thorough guide in *Back Surgery: Is It Right for You?* In my busy practice and at the top spinal research organizations where I have worked, I have seen patients agonizing over their decisions. I know there is a pressing need for comprehensive information about back problems and treatments. The explosion in the technology associated with the treatment of back problems in the last twenty years, and the corresponding growth in the number of available procedures, provide even more good reasons for you to turn to such a guide, since there has also been an explosion of inaccurate and misleading information.

I was shocked recently when I looked up "disc replacement" on an Internet search engine and saw the dizzying array of information that emerged. Even on sites for which I paid a fee, the material was confusing, and I could not decipher whether something was objective information or a veiled (biased) advertisement. Sites that touted the latest breakthroughs did not have them; the information often lagged behind a few years. But unless you have a medical degree, you probably would have no idea that the information you received was inaccurate, incomplete, or misleading. *Back Surgery: Is It Right for You?* painlessly cuts through the confusion.

The first thing you should know about your back is that the spine is the most complicated and delicate part of the body. In order for you to make an informed treatment decision (and prevent future troubles!), it is essential for you to understand your back and what might be causing your problem. That's why Part One of this book starts by taking a tour of your back to learn about its anatomy, from bones to ligaments to muscles. Equally helpful, I hope, will be the examination of your back's all-important function as the core of your body, which is crucial to movement and flexibility; as the protector of your nerves; and as the vital highway for information throughout your body.

Next, you will take a look at what might be causing your pain. There are typical categories into which most spine problems fit. Is your discomfort caused by arthritis, a traumatic injury, infection, everyday stress and strain, or another problem? This book will help you answer that question.

Nonsurgical options are the first treatments to consider. In recent years, there has been a dramatic increase in the introduction and use of new, effective drugs, including anti-inflammatory medications, pain medications, muscle relaxers, nerve stabilizers, steroids, and patches. In addition to drug therapy, you'll learn about physical and manipulation therapies, acupuncture, and pain management procedures.

Then you'll investigate your surgical choices, including benefits and risks. You'll take a thorough look at surgeries of the neck, also known as the cervical spine. You may have been presented with the option of cervical fusion, bone grafting, cervical foraminotomy, or cervical disc replacement, and we'll study each one. Perhaps your pain is in your lower back, in which case you'll be particularly interested in the discussion of surgeries of the lumbar spine. There are a number of surgeries from which to choose, including lumbar microdiscectomy, lumbar laminectomy, and lumbar fusion, all of which are offered in either traditional or minimally invasive versions.

If you do decide that back surgery is necessary, Part Two of this book will guide you along the way. First, you'll learn about preparing for surgery, including choosing your surgeon and care facility, and you'll find guidelines to help you get ready for either outpatient or inpatient surgery. This book, of course, also offers advice about your successful recovery, exploring what to expect immediately after your surgery, possible early complications, and physical therapy and rehabilitation.

Equally important is "A Healthy Back for Life," the last part of the book. In the hope that you can prevent future back problems, this book discusses how to keep your back strong, including safely using exercise to do so. You'll also learn about nutrition, which is key in the prevention of osteoporosis and in weight management—crucial for a healthy back, since excess weight stresses the back and is responsible for many ailments. And you will examine ergonomics, the study of equipment design that may prevent back problems. Ergonomics has become a buzzword in recent years, but it should be much more than that in your life. I hope that it will become a tool that you can put into practice everywhere—your home, your office, and your car.

Finally, an entire chapter is dedicated to back pain and personal psychology. For example, depression is a severe but common symptom of back pain, and I will help you understand its challenges. You will gain a better understanding of the pain and pain relief processes in your brain, as well. Knowing how the mind can both react to and resort to physical pain will make the healthful management of your back concerns even more successful.

I am certainly glad to accompany you on such an important journey. I, of course, can't single-handedly stop your pain, but I am delighted that *Back Surgery: Is It Right for You?* may be able to make what is often a highly stressful information-gathering and decision-making process virtually painless.

PART ONE

Deciding Whether Back Surgery Is for You

INTRODUCTION

How well do you know your own back—its structure, its strength, its fragility? Perhaps you recognize certain terms, such as *vertebrae* and *spinal cord,* from a biology class you took years ago. But chances are you can benefit immensely from a comprehensive review of the anatomy and function of the spine. When you have back pain, a limited concept of the spinal area is not enough. You need to understand the proper curvature of the spine, the areas where damage is most dire, and the "why" behind the pain associated with spinal arthritis, unhealthy discs, and injured ligaments—just to name a few of the disorders explained in this book. Chapters 1 and 2 will get you to that point of command.

The information doesn't stop there. Chapters 3 and 4 of *Back Surgery: Is It Right for You?* delve into various treatment options so that you can find resolution. People who suffer from back pain usually go for conservative, noninvasive treatments at first. Quite a few nonsurgical choices—such as medications, physical therapies, and muscle stretching—are explored in this book. But ultimately you, like countless others, might come to the decision that surgery is your best option for relief. So we will review various surgical procedures as well. You will feel much more prepared to make the optimal treatment decision after studying the details behind decompression surgeries and fusion surgeries, for example. Of course, we will look into the complications that could arise, but we will also focus on how the corrective measures of these surgeries can make your spine the functional, stable core that it was meant to be.

If you are feeling overwhelmed by all there is to learn, put your mind at rest. This book is specifically designed to give you information in small, organized doses. Use it as a reference book, a handbook, a companion. Read it with confidence, knowing you will be educated and therefore capable of holding a productive discussion with your health practitioner. Get ready to become an expert and your own advocate for a healthier, happier back.

1

Understanding Your Back

Trying to make a decision about back surgery without fully understanding the anatomy and function of your back is like attempting to drive a car to a faraway destination without a road map. In this chapter, we'll take a guided tour of your back. Then, we'll learn about the essential roles your back plays in your life as a house for your nerves, as your body's electrical signal highway, as your body's core, and as the key structure behind your ability to move and flex.

ANATOMY — TAKE A TOUR OF YOUR BACK

If you are like most people, you have probably always taken your back for granted. You may not even think of it as a discrete body part, like an arm or leg. Nothing, however, could be further from the truth. Your back is, in fact, one of the most complex, delicate, and essential parts of your body.

The *back* is a general term used to describe the spine and its surrounding muscles, as well as the nerves, discs, and bones that make up this complex structure. The word *spine* is not used uniformly, even in the medical community; I will use it to refer collectively to the bones, ligaments, muscles, nerves, and discs that constitute the back. I will use the term *spinal column* to indicate the bony architecture of the back—specifically, the tower of bony segments called *vertebrae*. Each vertebra is separated from the next by a *disc,* which acts like a cushion, and it is this structure that allows the spinal column to move. But it's the *spinal cord* that, along with your brain, makes up the central nervous system (CNS).

Spinal Cord

Just where does the spinal cord start? The spinal cord is like an extension cord of the brain. The lower part of the brain becomes the spinal cord and enters a canal—called the *spinal canal*—within the spinal column. The spinal cord and the spinal nerve roots reside within the spinal canal and are covered by a thin membrane called the *dura*. Actually, the dura covers the brain, the entire spinal cord, and the nerves before they exit the spine. The dura is like an envelope that keeps the fluid surrounding the nerves in place. This fluid is called the *cerebrospinal fluid* (CSF).

There are actually thirty-one pairs of spinal nerves that begin in the spinal cord. Therefore, the spinal cord can most simply be defined as a collection of nerve fibers. These fibers carry messages or impulses to and from the brain, allowing you to do everything from lifting your foot off a sharp piece of glass to smiling for the camera. The nerves are divided into major types—cervical, thoracic, lumbar, and sacral—and leave the spinal column at locations that are similarly named.

Sections of the Spine

There are four main sections to your spine: the cervical spine (neck), the thoracic spine (midback), the lumbar spine (lower back), and the sacrum/coccyx (pelvis). The cervical spine has seven bones. The first one is called C1, the second C2, and so forth. The first and second bones in the cervical spine are also called the *atlas* (C1) and the *axis* (C2). The thoracic spine has twelve bones. They are called T1, T2, T3, etc. The lumbar spine has five bones, which are larger than the other bones of the spine, since they carry much of the body weight. These are numbered L1 to L5. The sacrum and the coccyx are part of the pelvis and, for the sake of our discussion, can be regarded as one big bone at the lowest part of the spine.

If you look at a normal spine from front or back, it has a straight alignment from top to bottom. If you look at it from the side, however, you see that the spinal column is not a straight column of bones stacked on top of each other. In order to maintain flexibility and balance, each segment of the spine has a specific curvature. See Figure 1.1, on the next page.

The cervical spine and the lumbar spine are normally placed in *lordosis* (a curve with its concavity directed backward), while the thoracic

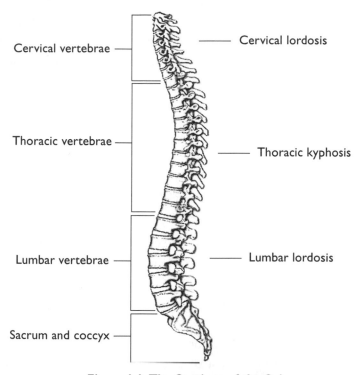

Cervical vertebrae —

—— Cervical lordosis

Thoracic vertebrae —

—— Thoracic kyphosis

Lumbar vertebrae —

—— Lumbar lordosis

Sacrum and coccyx —

Figure 1.1 The Sections of the Spine

spine is normally placed in *kyphosis* (a curve that is directed forward). Normal cervical lordosis and normal thoracic kyphosis are from twenty to forty degrees. In the lumbar spine, lordosis is normally thirty to fifty degrees. These curvatures are extremely significant. A change in the angles of these curves can occur for many reasons. In the cervical spine, *degenerative arthritis*—a process characterized by the degeneration (deterioration) of the cartilage, the formation of osteophytes (outgrowths of bone) in the joint, and inflammation—can lead to disc collapse and cause reversal of the normal lordosis into kyphosis. Fractures in the thoracic spine from *osteoporosis*—loss of bone tissue resulting in brittle bones—can increase the kyphosis curve, causing the humpback deformity that commonly affects senior citizens. Reversal of lordosis in the lumbar spine can occur because of the destruction of normal bone by a fracture, or by a disease like cancer. Loss of lordosis in the lumbar spine can result in *flat back syndrome,* which is a painful condition.

Flat back syndrome causes imbalance in the muscular structures of the lumbar spine. It was commonly seen after operations performed two or three decades ago, when the significance of lordosis in the lumbar spine was not appreciated by spine surgeons and the implants used in surgery did not allow doctors to maintain these curves of the spine. A very common implant used thirty years ago was the Harrington rod, which made the lower back very straight. There have been substantial improvements in the technology of implants over the years. Today we have implants that are strong and flexible, allowing your spine surgeon to maintain the curves of the back, even after surgery.

Cervical Spine

The *cervical spine*—the highest level of the spine—houses and protects the spinal cord as it leaves the skull. The cervical spine also supports the head and is involved in movements of the neck and the head, such as rotation, forward flexion, and backward extension. The axis (the second bone in the cervical spine, or C2) has an upward projection called the *dens*, which makes a second joint with the ring-shaped atlas (the first bone in the cervical spine, or C1), the structure upon which the skull sits. This joint is responsible for most of the rotation of the head, known as *atlanto-axial rotation*. See Figure 1.2 for a helpful illustration.

Most of the cervical vertebrae (C2-7) have small canals on either side. These canals, called the *transverse foramens*, house an artery called the *vertebral artery*. This artery is essential in supplying blood to parts of the brain. Again, refer to Figure 1.2.

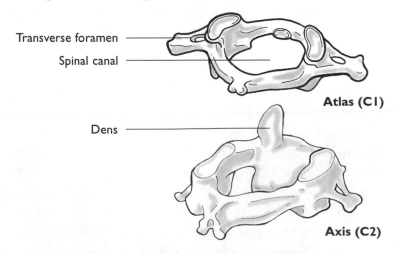

Figure 1.2 The Top of the Cervical Spine

The vertebrae, discussed and illustrated on pages 12 to 13, are connected by small joints called *facet joints*. On each side of the cervical vertebrae, between each facet joint, there is an area of bone called a *lateral mass*. This bony area is where spinal surgeons place screws when *fusion surgery*—the removal of an abnormal disc and the fusion of the surrounding vertebrae—is attempted from the rear of the cervical spine.

Injury to the spinal cord at the level of the cervical spine can be devastating or even deadly. The upper part of the spinal cord controls our breathing, and if a fracture places pressure over that area, we can stop breathing and potentially die as a result. The higher the injury, the worse its outcome. The lower the injury to the spinal cord, the more functions are preserved. A person who has an injury to the spinal cord at the C4 vertebra, for example, will not be able to breathe on his own. An injury at the C5 vertebra, by contrast, may allow the person to breathe and shrug his shoulders.

Thoracic Spine

The ribs attach in the front of the chest (anteriorly) to the breastbone (sternum), and in the back (posteriorly) to the thoracic vertebral bones. For this reason, the *thoracic spine* is very rigid (less mobile), as is the rib cage, which houses the heart and the lungs. The spinal cord in the area of the thoracic spine is essential for the functions of the lower body. Injury to the spinal cord at the level of the thoracic spine can lead to paralysis of the lower extremities and disorders of the bowel, bladder, and sexual functions.

At each level of the thoracic spine, a spinal nerve exits the spine and wraps around the rib cage. Any pressure on a nerve in the area (for example, from a disc herniation or a tumor) can result in pain that encircles the chest. This can lead to a false diagnosis of indigestion or a heart attack.

Problems in the thoracic spine are uncommon compared with those in the more mobile cervical and lumbar spines. *Disc herniations*—protruding or bulging discs—are common in the lumbar spine, for example, whereas in the thoracic spine they are rare.

Lumbar Spine

The *lumbar spine* is the lowest mobile section of the spinal column. It has five segments. Due to its mobility, the lumbar spine is subject to many problems, such as strains, disc herniations, and even fractures. The most common disc to degenerate (i.e., to deteriorate from wear and tear) and herniate is the L4-5 disc. The next most common disc to suffer from disc degeneration and herniation is the L5-S1 disc.

Sacrum/Coccyx

The *sacrum* and the *coccyx*—the latter of which is the remnant of a tail we used to have millions of years ago—constitute the lowest part of the spine. They are parts of the pelvis, which houses important structures such as the ovaries, the uterus, the bladder, and some of the abdominal contents.

The end of the spinal cord, called the *conus medullaris,* is located at the L1 or L2 vertebra. However, many spinal nerves continue to pass down along the spinal canal before exiting the spinal column. A collection of such spinal nerves distal to (lower than) the conus is called the *cauda equina.* It is located in the lumbosacral area. A massive disc herniation in this area can cause inability to control bowel and bladder functions. This condition is an emergency and is called *cauda equina syndrome.*

Vertebrae

The spinal column is made of many bony segments known as vertebrae, which maintain mobility and flexibility and provide protection to the nerves and the spinal cord. The vertebrae are similar in shape, but they vary in size according to the amount of weight they carry. Each vertebra within a section of the spine has a specific name and number. Your spine surgeon will usually localize a disc herniation using these designations. As previously mentioned, the most common level at which we encounter disc herniations is the L4-5 disc space. This simply means that the disc between the fourth lumbar (L4) vertebra and the fifth lumbar (L5) vertebra has herniated. A disc herniation in the neck is described in a similar manner. The most common level for a disc herniation in the neck is the C5-6 level. This refers to a disc herniation between the fifth cervical (C5) vertebra and the sixth cervical (C6) vertebra.

Each vertebra has a large, oval section in the front called the *vertebral body.* The rear (posterior) part of each vertebra has bony projections called *processes.* The *spinous process* is the fairly sharp, bony structure in the rear of the vertebra. If you touch the middle of your back, you can

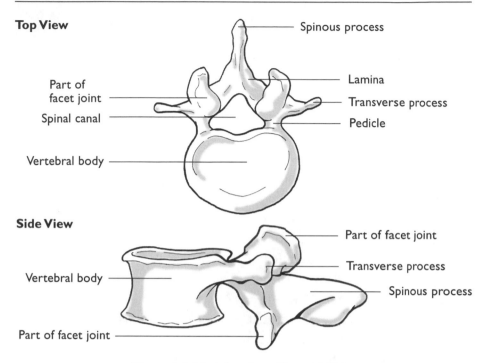

Top View

Spinous process

Part of facet joint

Lamina

Transverse process

Spinal canal

Pedicle

Vertebral body

Side View

Part of facet joint

Transverse process

Vertebral body

Spinous process

Part of facet joint

Figure 1.3 Vertebra from Top and Side

feel these projections. Only the vertebrae in the thoracic and the lumbar spine have *transverse processes*, which extend to the sides of the vertebrae. All of these features are illustrated in Figure 1.3.

The *lamina* is like the roof of the spinal canal. It is the bone to which some of the muscles over your spine attach. At the upper border of the lamina starts a cylindrical bony canal that connects the rear of the vertebra to the front. This bony canal is called the *pedicle*. The pedicles are very strong and make up the borders of the spinal canal.

As discussed, the vertebrae are connected by small joints called the facet joints, which give the spine flexibility. The facet joint, in the rear part of your spine, along with the disc in the front, allows some motion at each segment. The facet joint is similar to other joints in your body, like the knee or the shoulder. As in the case of these other joints, facet joints can be affected by arthritis, and, if arthritis occurs, these joints can place pressure on nerves and cause pain, numbness, or weakness. On magnetic resonance imaging (MRI) studies, a radiologist will call this *facet hypertrophy.* Other terms used to describe this condition are *facet syndrome* or *facet arthropathy.*

Discs

Many of the problems that occur in your spine stem from the *discs*. See Figure 1.4 for an illustration. Each disc, which is shaped like a miniature automobile tire, is situated in the front (anterior) of the spine, between two vertebral bodies, and acts as a cushion. The disc has an outer envelope called the *annulus*. Attached to the annulus are many small nerves that can transmit pain signals to the brain. The annulus is the part of the disc that is commonly injured, causing the common disorder known as *low back pain*, also called *discogenic pain*.

The inner part of the disc is called the *nucleus pulposus*. It has a softer consistency and can protrude outward through tears that occur in the annulus. This is commonly referred to as a *herniated disc, herniated nucleus pulposus*, or *HNP*. Unlike the annulus, the nucleus pulposus does not have any nerve endings. The nucleus causes problems when it herniates and places pressure on an adjacent nerve. Research has also shown that there are chemicals within the nucleus that can irritate a nerve by causing inflammation if they come into contact with it. If you have pain radiating from the spine, but the MRI does not show pressure on any nerves, you may be having pain caused by the chemicals that are released from the nucleus pulposus and not from pressure of the disc on the nerve root.

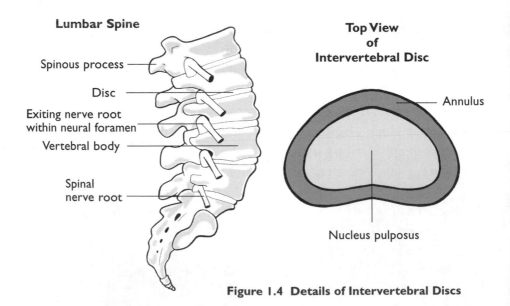

Figure 1.4 Details of Intervertebral Discs

Neural Foramen

The *neural foramen* is the tunnel through which the nerves leave the spinal column. See Figure 1.4 on page 14. It is made up of two half circles. The upper vertebra possesses one half of the circle and the lower vertebra possesses the other half. Put together, the two half circles of the tunnel make a canal through which the nerves pass out of the spinal column. The greater the distance between the two vertebrae, the larger the canal. The distance between the vertebrae depends on the height of the discs. Any process that decreases the height of the disc, such as degeneration or infection of the disc (discitis), can cause reduction in the diameter of the neural foramen, which in turn places pressure on the spinal nerve. This problem is known as *foraminal stenosis.* You can get foraminal stenosis from a disc bulge within the neural foramen, enlargement of the ligamentum flavum (see page 16), disc collapse, or arthritic enlargement of the facet joint. Any of these can produce pain, numbness, or weakness along the course of a particular nerve.

The plural of neural foramen is *neural foramina.* You will find both terms used throughout this book.

Ligaments

Ligaments are tough sheets of fibrous tissue that connect one bone to another. This connection makes our body resilient and strong, while allowing mobility and flexibility. If the force of an accident or fall is strong enough, ligaments can tear and, unfortunately, they don't heal as quickly as bones. Whiplash injuries involve damage to ligaments, which is why it takes a long time for pain from whiplash to go away.

Because there is little calcium in ligaments, they don't show up on X-ray studies. An MRI is a better test to check for damage to ligaments, but even an MRI does not show all ligament tears. The extent of the injury depends on the location of the damaged ligament and its function. If the ligament is very important, damage to it can cause abnormal movement between two bones, and this abnormal relationship of bones can sometimes be seen on an X-ray or CT (Computed Tomography) scan.

Figure 1.5 illustrates various spinal ligaments. One ligament that is very long and strong is the *anterior longitudinal ligament,* which is found

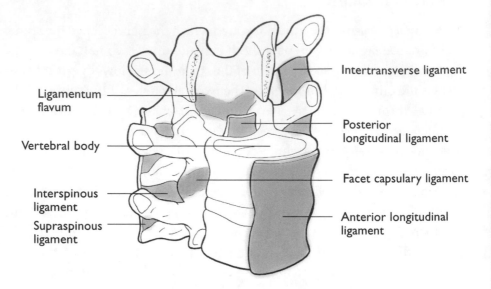

Intertransverse ligament

Ligamentum
flavum

Posterior
longitudinal ligament

Vertebral body

Facet capsulary ligament

Interspinous
ligament

Anterior longitudinal
ligament

Supraspinous
ligament

Figure 1.5 Spinal Ligaments

in front of the vertebral body. The anterior longitudinal ligament spans
from the neck to the pelvis. Another similar ligament is found in the
rear of the vertebral body and is called the *posterior longitudinal ligament.*
An important ligament inside the spinal canal, underneath the lamina,
is called the *ligamentum flavum.* The ligamentum flavum is also called
the yellow ligament because of its color. The *yellow ligament* is not continuous, like the posterior and anterior longitudinal ligaments, but it is
found at each level of the spine, where it maintains strong connections
between the bony vertebral segments. If you do have back surgery, your
surgeon will have to remove a small section of this ligament to see the
nerves that exit the spine. Removal of this small ligamentous section
will not have long-lasting effects and is a necessary part of the operation.
There are quite a few additional ligaments, some of which are labelled
in Figure 1.5 to show the complicated structure of the spine.

As we go down the spine, the ligaments get larger and stronger. The
ligaments in the pelvis are particularly strong, in order to support the
added weight they must bear. *Iliolumbar* and *lumbosacral ligaments* are
examples of these.

Muscles

The muscles surrounding your spine are important because they are the workhorses in moving your spine from one position to another. Three large muscles are found around your spine. They are called the *spinalis, longissimus,* and *iliocostalis* muscles. As a group, they are called the *erector spinae* muscle. See Figure 1.6 for a clearer understanding of these important features. These muscles are found in the mid- and lower back.

There are also muscles around the neck, which are much smaller than the erector spinae muscles. These muscles are injured much more readily than ligaments, since they are not as strong. But, just as they are injured quickly, they heal quickly, too; as we have noted, muscles heal faster and better than the ligaments around your spine.

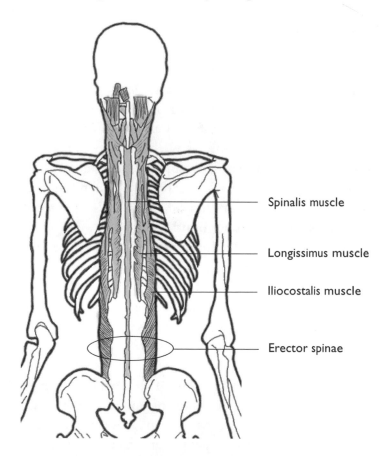

Spinalis muscle

Longissimus muscle

Iliocostalis muscle

Erector spinae

Figure I.6 Spinal Muscles

FUNCTION —
WHAT YOUR BACK CAN DO FOR YOU

We've defined your back and discussed its vital anatomy. Now let's put the pieces of the puzzle together. Just what does this complex part of the body do for you?

First, the brain processes all nerve impulses and disperses them throughout the body along the spinal cord, which is like a highway for nerve signals. The spinal cord is a collection of many nerves delicately intertwined, just like the lanes on the highway. The spinal nerves are similar to the exits on that highway. The anterior (front) side of the spinal cord passes information away from the brain and the posterior (rear) part of the spinal cord sends information toward the brain. Take, for example, a pleasurable foot massage. The sensation that your foot is being massaged gets transferred to the brain first by receptors in the skin of your foot, which receive the signals of touch and pressure. These receptors then transfer the information to the local nerves that relay this signal to your spinal cord. From there, the signal is transferred to the brain by other nerves in the rear part of your spinal cord.

Flexibility is also a key function of your spine. Your spine is flexible because the spinal column, as we have seen, is made of many separate bony vertebrae. The discs, facet joints, and ligaments hold the separate segments together and allow motion between them. In your everyday life, that flexibility means you can get in and out of a car, sit, stand, walk, and lift objects from the ground.

Without the spinal column, the spinal cord would also be very vulnerable. Furthermore, the spinal column acts as the main support beam to hold your body in place. Without it, your body would have no shape and you would not be able to stand. The spinal column maintains your posture and acts as an anchor for the muscles of your back.

*   *   *

Now that we've taken a tour of your back, in terms of both form and function, it will be much easier for you to understand your back problem. Is it arthritis, a traumatic injury, cancer, infection, a deformity, or just a strain from everyday wear and tear? We'll take a detailed look in the next chapter.

2

Determining the Cause of Your Back Problem

Sometimes the source of your back pain is evident. You are lucky enough to walk away from a car wreck, but your back is aching and you have a case of whiplash. Or you pick up a heavy storage box and immediately feel sharp pain. Other times, though, the source of the pain is a mystery. Where did it come from? Why doesn't it stop!

Before you make decisions about how to relieve your pain, you need to identify and understand it. In this chapter, we'll examine all types of spine problems. First, we'll take a look at the most frequent culprit—arthritis—in causing conditions such as herniated discs. Then it's on to traumatic injuries, including sprains and strains, fractures, and dislocations. Finally, we'll study other health problems such as cancer, and deformities like scoliosis, that can cause distress.

ARTHRITIS

Arthritis is responsible for most back problems. That is because arthritis is extremely common. As mentioned in Chapter 1, arthritis is a process characterized by the degeneration of the cartilage, the formation of osteophytes (outgrowths of bone) in the joint, and inflammation. It's important to understand the process of degeneration in detail. When you are an infant and a child, the tissues in your body have a high water content—as high as 97 percent. As you age, your body slowly loses water, the depletion of which can be seen in the discs as well as in the cartilage in the joints. This is analogous to the process through which a grape turns into a raisin; as fruits lose water, they shrink and become wrinkled. Similarly, as your body slowly loses water content over time, your skin wrinkles, your bones form irregular projections called osteophytes, the discs in your spine shrink and become stiff, and so forth.

As the water content of the discs decreases, their color changes on MRI images and you may hear your doctor say that you have a "black disc." Synonymous terms that your spinal specialist may use are *internal disc derangement* and *degenerative disc disease.* This condition can—but does not always—cause back pain.

DISC HERNIATION

As I look at MRI studies with my patients, they often ask me, "How many bad discs do I have?" I usually tell them that, even though many discs in their spine may look abnormal, they are probably functioning well and are not necessarily causing pain. For this reason, we don't treat our patients based on the MRI results, but based on their complaints and symptoms. Several important research studies showed that if we pick one hundred people over the age of sixty who have no problems with their backs, and get MRIs of their spines, we would see that more than half of them have degenerated discs or disc herniations. This demonstrates that we don't have to worry about every abnormality that we see on a diagnostic study. We have to judge the significance of any abnormality based on the symptoms it causes. As with any rule, there are exceptions to this one, too. If your doctor detects signs of cancer or osteoporosis, treatment should not be delayed, even if you have no symptoms.

Disc herniations can be a consequence of degenerative disc disease or arthritis in the spine. As the disc degenerates, the outer covering, also called the annulus, becomes incompetent and allows the nucleus of the disc, also called the nucleus pulposus, to herniate outward toward an exiting nerve root. This herniation can place pressure on the nerve, on the spinal cord, or both. If the disc herniation does not come into contact with a nerve, you may feel only back pain, without any pain in your legs or arms. On the other hand, if a disc herniation places pressure on a nerve or on the spinal cord, you can also feel numbness, weakness, or tingling in the arms or legs.

A disc herniation will cause the most severe pain in the first few weeks. If you are experiencing this, you know it is like having a knife stuck in your arm. The majority of people who suffer from a disc herniation will have substantial improvement in their pain within three months, without surgery. Since the symptoms of disc herniations often do improve after a few weeks or months, some researchers wanted to see if the size of a disc herniation actually decreases over time. They performed MRI studies on patients who had disc herniations and then they repeated the MRI studies two years later. They saw that the size of a disc herniation does decrease over time in most people.

There are different ways of describing the configuration of the herniation. In order of increasing severity, they are: disc bulge, disc protrusion, and disc extrusion. A *disc bulge* is a good description of what is seen on the MRI and is usually very small. A *disc protrusion* is a type of disc herniation in which a piece of the disc has moved out of place, but is still attached to the main part of the disc. An *extruded disc*, which is usually larger than a bulge, is a piece of disc that has lost contact with the main part of the disc. This type of disc herniation can be very large, even compressing a few nerves.

One of the most common questions that your spine specialist will ask you is whether you have leg pain (or arm pain), back pain, or both. The answer to this question is very important, since it will guide your treatment plan. Pain concentrated in your lower back or neck is called *midline axial pain*. Axial pain can be caused by many different problems, which can include arthritis, fractures, cancer, deformity, or other, less common problems. Pain mostly in your legs or arms is called *extremity pain, radiating pain,* or *radiculopathy.* Some spine specialists prefer to use the terms *mechanical* (i.e., axial) versus *nonmechanical* (i.e., radiating) *pain.*

The location of your pain, its intensity, and the presence or absence of associated numbness, weakness, or tingling are the most important factors that your doctor will consider. Most patients are too agitated by their pain to differentiate between leg (or arm) and back pain. Often, patients have both, and they need some guidance in determining exactly where their pain is. Pain that originates in the spine can be diffuse and deep (which makes it hard to pinpoint), as compared with pain in the extremities, which is usually sharp and localized. Remember, if you have radiating pain in your leg or arm, the problem usually originates in your back, and your back needs treatment, not your extremity.

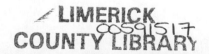

A disc herniation is usually easily diagnosed by a routine MRI. In some cases, the MRI may not be clear and your surgeon may consider having a CT-myelogram performed as an additional diagnostic study. A myelogram uses X-ray and a contrast media (dye) to visualize the spinal canal, spinal cord, and nerves. In a CT-myelogram, the myelogram is followed by a CT scan, whose cross-sectional images reveal information about the bony structures of the spine. Together, these tests provide images of both bone and nerves, and can therefore be very useful in diagnosing your disc problem.

Neurodiagnostic studies such as electromyography (EMG) and nerve conduction studies can also be obtained to evaluate the function of the nerves affected by a disc herniation. An electromyography is an electrical study that measures the response of muscle to the stimulation of a nerve. A variation of this test is the nerve conduction velocity (NCV), which measures the speed of signal transport within the nerve.

Cervical Disc Herniation

Just like the parts of an automobile, the sections of the spine that are involved in more motion are susceptible to more injury, wear, and break-down. Discs that are more mobile lose hydration faster. For this reason, they degenerate more quickly than ones that do not move as much. If a disc loses its hydration, it can bulge, much as the tire of a car bulges from the sides as it loses air. This bulging can place pressure on a nerve, which can result in pain, numbness, or weakness. The lower part of the neck is more mobile than the upper part and, as a result, more disc her-niations occur there. Disc herniations are more commonly seen at the C4-5, C5-6, and C6-7 level.

Each nerve in the cervical spine corresponds to a specific area of skin on the arm and the hand. For example, the C6 nerve exits between the C5 and C6 vertebrae and supplies sensation to the hand in the area of the thumb and the index finger. The C7 nerve exits between the C6 and C7 vertebrae and is responsible for sensation over the long finger. The C8 nerve exits the spine between the C7 and T1 vertebrae and is respon-sible for sensation over the ring and little fingers. If you are experienc-ing numbness and pain radiating from the neck to the first, second, and third fingers, your doctor will be looking for a disc herniation on the MRI at the level of the C5-6 or the C6-7 level.

Just as each nerve provides sensation to different areas of your arm, each nerve conducts signals to specific muscles. By discovering which muscle is weak, your spine specialist can determine which nerve is the source of your problem. For example, the C5 nerve is responsible for conducting signals to the biceps and deltoid muscles. These muscles provide power for elbow flexion and shoulder elevation. The C6 nerve is mainly responsible for wrist extension. The C7 nerve is responsible for elbow extension, wrist flexion, and extension of the fingers. The C8 nerve is responsible for opening and closing the fingers and making a fist.

If a disc herniates in your neck and places pressure on your spinal cord, it can cause problems with walking, balance, and coordination. This condition, called *myelopathy*, is different from a disc herniation that places pressure on a specific nerve, which is called *radiculopathy*. Myelopathy can cause difficulty changing direction when you are walking or clumsiness in your hands, such as trouble buttoning your shirt or a tendency to drop dishes you are washing. Sometimes, handwriting changes occur. At times, these symptoms are accompanied by pain, but pain from myelopathy is usually vague and poorly characterized.

Normally, as you move your arm, the nerves that run from the neck through the arm also move and stretch. A disc herniation in the neck can limit the movement of the nerves as you move your arm. The nerves are under the least tension when you hold your arm above your head, which can decrease your symptoms. I have even seen people driving with one arm placed on their head, and I immediately recognize the type of back problem these people have!

The most difficult symptom of a herniated disc is pain. It is usually accompanied by numbness and weakness, which is less bothersome to most people but is worrisome to your spine specialist. This is because weakness is more difficult to treat than pain. Weakness that is present for more than three months may cause atrophy of muscles, which need stimulation to maintain power and size. The lack of this stimulation over a period of time may cause irreversible damage. For this reason, your spine specialist may offer a more aggressive treatment plan when weakness is present.

Making the Most of Your Consultation

Don't go to your consultation with the idea that your spine surgeon can find your problem just by looking at your MRI. The information from the MRI is secondary to the history you provide, which is the most important part of your evaluation.

Most spine specialists will try to maximize the benefit you get from your office visit. You also have to remember, however, that the time you have available with your spine surgeon is not unlimited. Most good spine surgeons are busy and devote only a portion of their time to patient evaluations. Their remaining time is devoted to surgery. Attempt to maximize your own benefit from this office visit by providing as much concise, accurate information as you can to help the spine surgeon find the origin of your problem.

Try to avoid descriptions such as, "Everything hurts." This will not help your cause in any way and can actually frustrate your doctor. Also avoid responses such as, "It hurts really bad." Again, this does not provide any useful information and can actually be counterproductive. Your specialist should be seeking information regarding the specific location and intensity of your pain, the presence or absence of any numbness, and the extent of weakness if it is present. Try to convey your message by explaining the changes in your life that the pain has caused. For example, "My arm pain is so bad that it wakes me up at night." Or, "My pain is so bad that I can no longer drive my car." This will put the intensity of your pain in perspective and will help your doctor devise the most appropriate treatment plan for your condition.

Lumbar Disc Herniation

Your lower back is also at risk for a disc herniation. This can cause numbness, weakness, and pain from the lower back all the way down to the toes. As we have reviewed, the disc can bulge like a car's tire, or it can have a tear that allows the center of the disc to herniate out into the spinal canal. Your symptoms will vary depending on the size and, most important, the location of the herniation. A small disc bulge can cause aching pain down the leg; a large disc herniation, however, can cause severe weakness and excruciating pain. Usually the pain from a lumbar disc herniation will worsen after you start walking, and your main complaint may be difficulty walking more than five minutes.

Patients frequently ask me about the size of their lumbar disc herniation, but the location of the herniation is usually more important than its size. One location of interest involves the neural foramina, which we discussed in Chapter 1 (see page 15). This is the tunnel that the nerve goes through to leave the spinal column, and it is just slightly larger than the nerve itself. The outer part of a disc forms one wall of this tunnel, so even a relatively small disc bulge within the neural foramina can cause many problems with the nerve. On the other hand, a large disc herniation that does not come in contact with a nerve may not cause any problems.

If a herniated disc places pressure on a nerve in the lumbar spine, it can result in pain traveling from the lower back down the leg. This is commonly called *sciatica* because it causes pain along the sciatic nerve, which is in fact a collection of nerves that runs from the lower back into the middle of the buttocks and then passes through the rear part of the thigh down to the feet. Around the knee, the nerves divide again, providing sensation to the various parts of the foot.

As in the neck, where each nerve provides sensation to part of the hand or arm, each nerve that exits the lumbar spine provides sensation to a specific part of the leg or foot. The S1 nerve furnishes sensation to the back of the leg, as well as the outer and bottom part of the foot. The L2 and L3 nerves supply sensation to the thigh, the L4 nerve to the inner parts of the leg and foot, and the L5 nerve to the front part of the leg and the top of the foot. So numbness on the top part of the foot corresponds to problems with the L5 nerve. Nerves also conduct signals for muscle movement. For example, the L4 nerve is responsible for elevation of the foot at the ankle joint, and the L5 nerve for elevation of the toes and the foot.

Your spine specialist should be asking you about precise areas of numbness. This can provide information about the specific disc that is placing pressure on a nerve. A disc herniation can occur at one, two, three, or more levels simultaneously. All parts of the story should fit together: the details of the MRI pictures, the distribution of your pain, and the physical examination. Variations to this scheme exist, and that is why you should rely on the experience and knowledge of your spine specialist to recognize these differences. The ability to recognize and make sense of the small details sets apart a good physician from a less knowledgeable one.

SPINAL STENOSIS

Another common condition of the spine is *spinal stenosis,* which can occur in the cervical or lumbar spine. Spinal stenosis involves the narrowing of the central spinal canal. Imagine a highway with five lanes that allow the traffic to flow relatively quickly, and then compare it with a section of the same highway that becomes two lanes; you can easily see the slowing of the cars. This is similar to what happens in spinal stenosis. As compared to a disc herniation, which usually affects a single nerve, spinal stenosis often affects multiple nerves and develops over a long period of time.

Spinal stenosis is usually easily diagnosed with an MRI. A myelogram can also be used to diagnose spinal stenosis. For more information on diagnoses and consultations, see the boxed inset titled "Making the Most of Your Consultation," on page 24.

Spinal stenosis can originate with arthritis and is usually seen in older patients. As we mentioned earlier, dehydration of the discs comes with age and arthritis, and it causes bulging of the disc inside the spinal canal. This causes a very small abnormal movement between each vertebra, also called *abnormal micromotion.* To compensate for this abnormal micromotion, the ligamentum flavum, which is inside the spinal canal, gets thicker. The facet joints also get bigger and place further pressure on the nerves within the spinal canal. The combination of the disc bulge, the ligamentum flavum thickening, and the enlargement of the facet joints is the cause of spinal stenosis.

Cervical Spinal Stenosis

Cervical spinal stenosis is less common than lumbar spinal stenosis. The symptoms are different, since, in the neck, not only are the nerves placed under pressure, but the spinal cord as well. As I mentioned, pressure on the spinal cord is called myelopathy and it can cause dull, aching pain. If you have cervical spinal stenosis, you can have imbalance when walking, along with pain radiating to your arms. Other symptoms may be clumsiness in the hands and lack of coordination. Changes in handwriting is another common complaint.

Arthritis is not the only process that can cause spinal stenosis in the neck. Even though cervical spinal stenosis is much more common in the elderly, it can also occur in younger people who are born with smaller spinal canals. Calcification of the posterior longitudinal ligament can cause similar symptoms. This is also called *OPLL*, which stands for Ossification of Posterior Longitudinal Ligament. Symptoms are similar to those resulting from arthritic spinal stenosis.

Lumbar Spinal Stenosis

One symptom of lumbar spinal stenosis is difficulty walking, including a feeling of heaviness in the legs after only a short distance. Sitting will usually improve the symptoms of spinal stenosis. This is because sitting causes tightening and thinning of the ligamentum flavum. This in turn makes the spinal canal a little bigger and reduces the symptoms until you stand up or start walking again. You may also find some relief by walking with a bent posture, as some people would do in the supermarket when pushing a cart. You may think it's the support provided by the cart that allows you to walk more comfortably, but it is actually the bent posture you assume that enables you to walk for longer periods. Sleeping in a straight position can cause more pain, and you may find yourself resting in the bent fetal position. Even though most people with spinal stenosis can walk for only a few minutes, they can often ride a bicycle for a long time. That's because your spine is placed in a bent posture when riding a bicycle.

SPONDYLOLYSIS AND SPONDYLOLISTHESIS

Before we get any further, I must go over some terms that can be very confusing. When diagnosing your back problem, your spinal specialist may talk about spondylo*sis*, spondylo*lysis*, or spondylo*listhesis*. Even though these terms sound similar, they refer to very different processes that can occur in your spine. The term *spondylosis* refers to degenerative changes, or arthritis of the spine. In contrast, the term *spondylolysis* refers to a stress fracture in the back of the spine. Specifically, this happens in the outer aspect of the lamina, usually because of a traumatic injury or a congenital condition. The term *spondylolisthesis* refers to the slippage of one vertebra over another.

So, when you hear the term *spondylosis*, you'll know it refers to degenerative changes or arthritis of the spine. Let's take a closer look at spondylolysis and spondylolisthesis.

Spondylolysis

Again, spondylolysis is a crack or fracture of the bone in the rear of a vertebra. This condition usually develops because of a fall during the teen years or repetitive backward bending of the type done by gymnasts and football players. Sometimes, however, spondylolysis is congenital or its causes are unknown. In most people, it goes unnoticed because it does not cause pain or dysfunction. Occasionally it is diagnosed because it causes pain when the patient bends backward. It commonly causes arthritis in one specific section of the lumbar spine and may result in spondylolisthesis, discussed next. Even though spondylolysis is seen in many patients with spondylolisthesis, not all people who have spondy-lolysis will develop slippage of the bone.

If you have spondylolysis, a high-quality CT scan or a bone scan is often the best diagnostic study. In this case, an MRI is not superior to the CT scan. If your spine surgeon has a high suspicion of spondylolysis, but can't see it on an MRI or a CT scan, she may decide to order a Single Photon Emission Computed Tomography (SPECT) scan, which can diagnose it more reliably than other tests. A SPECT scan is a very specialized test that is usually done in the department of nuclear medicine of a hospital.

Spondylolisthesis

To visualize the concept of spondylolisthesis, imagine a stable tower of perfectly stacked books. If one of the books from the bottom of the tower begins to slide, the entire stack will start moving, and soon the whole pile may become unstable. Spondylolisthesis is such a slippage, and it can be caused by spondylolysis, arthritis, fracture, or a congenital abnor-mality. Spondylolisthesis is seen commonly in gymnasts, ballet dancers, heavy weight lifters, and football players who have spondylolysis. The most common type of spondylolisthesis is degenerative or arthritic. If you have spondylolisthesis, you may hear your doctor refer to the L5-S1 part of your spine. What she means is that the L5 vertebra is slipping over the S1 vertebra.

Once a slip occurs, it may not necessarily get worse. Many patients have a small slip (grade I) that will remain as it is, without worsening, for the rest of their lives. Not all patients with spondylolisthesis have pain, and so not all will need any treatment. But for some, as one bone slips over the other, the nerves can become entangled between the bones, which may cause neurologic difficulties such as weakness, numbness, or pain.

Remember, not all slips get worse. Not all slips need surgery. Not all slips are painful. The pain from most slips improves with conservative treatment. However, the slip does not go back to the original configuration once it occurs. The best way to treat the pain is to keep the back muscles strong, which can compensate for the weak bony architecture.

There are four categories of slippage that can be detected by X-ray. Grade I represents the smallest slip and grade IV is the worst. If the slip is substantial, it can easily be seen on X-rays, but more subtle slippages can be difficult to identify. If you have pain from spondylolisthesis, your doctor may order an MRI to evaluate the severity of the slip and the condition of the nerves.

TRAUMATIC INJURIES

One day your spine is fine, the next you are sidelined by pain. The cause is no mystery: whether you fell off a ladder and seriously hurt your spinal cord or slightly damaged soft tissue in a minor car accident, you've been injured and you need help. Let's take a look at these types of traumatic injuries.

Sprains, Strains, and Whiplash

Sprains are injuries to the ligaments and *strains* are injuries to the muscle tissue. *Whiplash* is an injury to soft tissue in the neck—muscles, tendons, or ligaments—from a sudden, unexpected force exerted on the head. Your spine specialist may call these injuries by other names, such as acceleration injury, whiplash injury, whiplash syndrome, cervical sprain syndrome, or hyperextension injury. If a bone is broken from a sudden movement of the head and neck, this injury is no longer called whiplash and is simply called a cervical spine fracture.

One reason these types of back problems are so prevalent is that there are so many ligaments and muscles in the neck that can be injured.

A car accident is often the culprit. When you sit in a car traveling at forty miles per hour, you, of course, are also moving at that same speed. If the car suddenly stops or decreases its speed because of an accident, your body will continue to move at the original speed. Since your head is relatively heavy and is attached to the mobile neck, the result will be a forward thrust of your head and neck. As the ligaments and the muscles in the rear of your neck tighten, your neck will then be thrown backward. As the neck violently jerks forward and backward, the muscles and the ligaments can be injured.

The neck pain that results from whiplash is often described as an aching sensation, which can be sharp or dull, and gets worse with movement. The pain can also be felt between the shoulder blades and in the arms. Usually, it becomes worse two or three days after the initial injury. Most people feel much better two weeks later and, by three months, the majority of people are back to normal. Unfortunately, 25 percent of people will have chronic pain and about 10 percent will have pain they describe as severe.

The diagnosis of whiplash injury is usually made from the history of the injury itself. A whiplash injury can result in a great deal of pain with no objective findings on diagnostic studies. MRI studies can rule out other, more serious, injuries, but the injury to the muscle tissue and the ligaments in the neck may be difficult to visualize on an MRI.

Fractures

As we discussed in Chapter 1, your back has a number of essential functions: to protect your nerves, allow mobility, and maintain the shape of your body. When a fracture occurs, it can affect all three functions. In addition, most fractures cause pain. Foremost on your mind may be the reduction of your pain. The more important reasons to treat fractures, however, are to avoid further nerve injury, worsening of deformity, and long-term disability. In general, as I have mentioned, fractures to the neck are much more dangerous than fractures of the lower back. This is because the spinal cord ends approximately at the level of the L1 vertebra, and fractures below that level don't usually cause paralysis, whereas in the neck, the spinal cord is vulnerable, making paralysis a risk.

Odontoid Fractures

Fractures of the *odontoid*—a projection of the second cervical vertebra that articulates with the first cervical vertebra—are a common type of fracture of the neck and usually result from falls or car accidents. Most fractures of the odontoid do not cause nerve damage or injury to the spinal cord. If you have a fracture to the middle part of the neck, it could be a simple fracture that will not cause neurologic problems and looks stable on X-rays, or it could be a more severe fracture associated with massive disc herniations or even dislocations of the facet joints.

Your spine surgeon may choose to obtain an MRI study or a CT scan. MRI studies provide more information about ligaments, nerves, and discs. A CT scan will provide more information about the configuration of the bony fracture and can show if a piece of bone was pushed into the spinal canal. Ordering both tests may be appropriate and should not be regarded as redundant.

Compression Fractures

A *compression fracture*, also called *osteoporosis insufficiency fracture*, is the most common fracture in the midback, but it can also occur in the lower back. The term describes a compression of the vertebral body, which is the bulky, oval, bony part of the vertebra in each bony segment. Up to the age of thirty, our body keeps absorbing calcium to make stronger bones. After that, we slowly lose calcium from our bones, and, as we get older, some of us have very weak bones that can break easily. This is why compression fractures are most common among senior citizens and can result from minor trauma or even simple lifting. They often cause a lot of pain, but do not ordinarily cause nerve damage or instability. The pain usually improves within six weeks.

Compression fractures can usually be easily diagnosed with routine X-rays. If the fracture is subtle, however, it may be difficult to see on an X-ray. In this case, if your doctor still suspects a compression fracture, an MRI can be a very sensitive test to detect this type of injury. A CT scan is a good way to evaluate the severity of the fracture. A CT scan will also determine whether any bone fragments have entered the spinal canal, endangering the spinal cord.

Burst Fractures

Mid- and lower back fractures usually result from a severe car accident or a fall from a height and are called *burst fractures*. Even though these fractures can be seen in the elderly, they are much more common in younger patients who are more often the victims of traumatic accidents and falls. In the midback, the ribs attach to the side of the vertebrae, protecting them from fractures. Because of this, much greater force is required to cause a fracture in the midback. But when such a fracture does happen, it can cause paralysis of the legs.

To diagnose this severe type of fracture, a CT scan is the favored test among spine surgeons. There are usually some bone fragments in the spinal canal, which the CT scan will reveal. An MRI can be used to obtain more information about any soft tissue injury such as nerve root compression or a ligament tear.

Dislocations

You have probably heard of a dislocated shoulder, or known someone who has had one. A *dislocation* is a disruption of the normal alignment of a joint. Facet joints can dislocate just like shoulders. As we discussed in Chapter 1, facet joints are small joints in the rear of the spine. Most commonly, facet dislocations are seen in the neck as the result of a severe accident. Facet dislocations can cause nerve injuries and they should be put back into place as soon as possible.

An X-ray is the first step in diagnosing this condition. A CT scan will show the dislocation if the X-ray is not clear. An MRI should be performed to evaluate injury to the spinal cord, the disc, and the nerves in that spinal segment.

A joint *subluxation* is a condition of instability in a joint that has not dislocated. Chiropractors and spine surgeons disagree on the use of the term *subluxation,* which is commonly used by chiropractors. Most spine surgeons don't use this term, since the condition can't reliably be seen during surgery or on diagnostic studies. Most likely, if you have been diagnosed with a subluxation, you suffer from muscle spasms that may improve with chiropractic manipulation.

CANCER

Cancer refers to the abnormal growth of cells that disrupts function and structures of body organs. If left unchecked, it can result in destruction of organs and even death. Cancers of the spine are rare. The most common cancer of the spine is one that has metastasized (spread) to the spine from other parts of the body. The spine is fertile ground for this, since it is rich in blood vessels that can transport cancerous cells. In men, prostate cancer can spread to the spine. In women, breast cancer can do the same. Lung cancer is another common type of cancer that can spread to the spine. Cancers that develop in the spine itself and don't spread are called *benign cancers*. They are usually small and don't grow over time. Aggressive cancers, by contrast, are usually large, grow fast, and invade nearby organs. There are many cancers and each one has a different characteristic, behavior, and prognosis.

Diagnosing the many cancers that can attack the spine ranges from easy to very difficult. A variety of tests is used to determine whether cancer is present and what type of cancer it is. These include bone scans, MRIs, CT scans, PET scans, myelograms, and blood tests.

INFECTION

Like cancer, infection of the spine is uncommon. However, it is certainly possible. An infection of the bone is called *osteomyelitis.* There are several reasons that your spine can get infected. If your immune system is weak or if you recently had surgery, your chances of getting an infection of the spine are much higher. Other conditions that raise your chances of getting a spine infection are diabetes and HIV infection. In children, who have extensive blood supply to the bone, infections of the bone are more common, usually arising from other body parts and spread by the circulation of the blood. An infection of the discs can also occur, and in that case, the infection is called *discitis.*

Moreover, infections can occur in the epidural space—the area between the dura, which is the outer covering of the spinal cord, and the bone. An infection in the epidural space can be devastating and must be treated immediately to avoid neurologic damage or even death. Symptoms usually include a rapid worsening of back pain and neurological problems. Appetite changes, general weakness, and fever are other common symptoms of infection of the spine.

Tuberculosis is a type of infection that can affect the lungs, the kidneys, or the bone in your spine. When the bone of the spine is infected with tuberculosis, it's called *Pott's disease.* This type of infection was common many years ago, but became less prevalent with the appropriate use of antibiotics. Unfortunately, with increased rates of HIV infection, Pott's disease has once again become more common.

Osteomyelitis of the spine and discitis can be diagnosed with an MRI study. *Bone scans* and *gallium scans* are other diagnostic tools your spine specialist can use to identify a spinal infection. These are nuclear scanning tests in which a radioactive marker is injected into a vein. After time is allowed for the bones to absorb the marker, a special camera takes images of the patterns of absorption by the bones. These images will indicate areas of inflammation, which could indicate an infection.

DEFORMITY

Deformity—whether it's something you have dealt with your whole life or just recently had to face—may be what's brought you, or is about to bring you, to your spine specialist's office. Let's take a look at two common deformities: scoliosis and kyphosis.

Scoliosis

Scoliosis is a curve of the spine. It is most often noted in the irregularly developing spines of teens. It's important to screen for scoliosis because it can worsen as the adolescent grows into adulthood. The fastest progression of the curve occurs when the teenager goes through the growth spurt of puberty. Once the child reaches her final height, the curve usually stops getting worse. Generally, in adolescent patients, curves of less than twenty degrees are observed. More severe curves are seen in children with other associated problems such as osteogenesis imperfecta (a congenital disorder causing fragile bones and consequent fractures), cerebral palsy, or paraplegia. When a curve becomes severe, it can cause breathing problems, frequent lung infections, difficulty sitting, and even death. Fortunately, severe curves are rare.

Adolescent scoliosis is usually detected by school screening programs. If the child has not reached her final height, she should be examined with an X-ray every six months to follow the progression of the curve. A spine specialist or a radiologist can measure the extent of the curve on an X-ray. X-rays are also the simplest and most reliable way to diagnose scoliosis in adults.

In adults and the elderly, arthritis, fractures, or tumors can cause scoliosis. Even though scoliosis can cause back pain, this pain does not develop quickly. Many times patients think that their scoliosis is the cause of their pain, but if pain develops quickly, it should not be blamed on scoliosis that has been there for many years.

Kyphosis

Kyphosis is the medical term for humpback deformity. Many mothers bring their children to doctors' offices asking for a checkup because their child has a pronounced curve of the back or bad posture. Many of these mothers themselves have this curve, too, since it is hereditary. This problem is called postural kyphosis, and it can improve with exercise and muscle strengthening.

X-rays are the best way to diagnose kyphosis in both children and adults. Kyphosis can also occur in the elderly because of the poor bone density that causes compression fractures. This disorder can be so pronounced that the head may not be raised up. In most cases, it is not correctable in the elderly.

*   *   *

Now that you are armed with the knowledge of precisely what your back problem is, whether it's from arthritis, a traumatic injury, cancer, or deformity, it's time to examine your options. In the next two chapters, we'll take a hard look at your choices. First, we'll examine the nonsurgical options, including medication, physical therapy, acupuncture, and pain management procedures. Then, it's on to a detailed assessment of surgical alternatives for both the neck and the lower back, including a thorough examination of both benefits and risks.

3

Nonsurgical Treatment Options

Conservative treatment is a term commonly used by spine specialists, referring to nonsurgical options. It should be regarded as a relative concept that compares one treatment method to another, more aggressive, one. Naturally, conservative treatment may not be the best option in every case, and you should examine all your choices before proceeding. Most doctors, however, will first use conservative treatments to resolve back problems. These treatments are usually less risky, though often not as effective, as more aggressive options, such as surgery. Imagine yourself on a ladder where the more conservative treatment options are at the bottom and the more aggressive options are at the top. In most cases you should start with the more conservative options and move up the ladder to the more aggressive ones, if necessary.

At the bottom of this ladder, you will find treatment options such as medications, stretching, heat and cold therapy, aquatherapy, physical therapy, massage therapy, acupuncture, and chiropractic treatments. As you climb the ladder with your spine specialist, you will encounter pain management procedures such as epidural injections, facet blocks, selective nerve blocks, and rhizotomy. Higher on the ladder, you will find minimally invasive surgical procedures, including microdiscectomy and a variety of decompression procedures. The most aggressive surgical procedures, at the top of the ladder, including fusion operations, are used for patients who have exhausted all other, more conservative, treatment options.

MEDICATIONS

Most people will use medications at some point to relieve their back pain. Even if you have decided to go ahead with surgery, you are probably taking some type of medication to reduce pain and increase function. There are different classes of medications and many different types of medications placed in various categories. In most cases, the medications within a category have similar benefits and side effects. Your doctor will guide you to the appropriate use of these medications and the interaction of one medication with another.

Anti-Inflammatory Drugs

The most common category of medications that your spine specialist may suggest is anti-inflammatory medications, which are divided into two groups: steroidal anti-inflammatory medications and nonsteroidal anti-inflammatory drugs, commonly called NSAIDs. Many NSAIDs have been approved by the Food and Drug Administration, including Arthrotec, Naprosyn, Voltaren, Indocin, Feldene, Clinoril, Motrin, Advil, Ibuprofin, Orudis, Ansaid, Lodine, Daypro, Oruvail, Toradol, Relafen, and Mobic. The basic effect they have on your body is similar, however: they reduce inflammation and swelling, which are the causes of the pain.

Your body has natural mechanisms both to cause and to fight inflammation. You can consider inflammation your friend as well as your enemy, since it is a process that summons white blood cells to the rescue in cases of infections, fractures, lacerations, or even cancer. Unfortunately, inflammation is also a major cause of pain. If you have arm or leg pain that is caused by a herniated disc in your neck or lower back, for example, it is most likely caused by pressure being placed on a nerve, resulting in inflammation in the area. This inflammation causes swelling of the nerve. That, in turn, results in more pressure from the disc. This creates a vicious cycle of more inflammation, along with more swelling and increased pain, which may ultimately result in numbness and weakness. In this case, inflammation is your foe and anti-inflammatory medications are your weapon. The downside of anti-inflammatory medication, however, is that it does not remove the cause of the problem, but only treats its effects.

Side effects are common to all anti-inflammatory medications. Gastritis and sudden gastric bleeding are the most common ones. This is because anti-inflammatory medications block chemicals that are produced in your stomach lining to protect you from gastritis and gastric bleeding. A common recommendation is to take the anti-inflammatory medications with food. This usually reduces the risks of gastric ulcers. Another method of fighting gastric ulcers is to take medications that reduce acids within your stomach. This, however, requires you to take a second pill to counteract the effects of the first one.

Cox-2 inhibitors, such as Celebrex and Vioxx, are a special class of NSAIDs that have a better safety profile for stomach ulcers and gastritis. They were approved a few years ago and became one of the most popular medications around. Unfortunately, after those medications were released, questions arose regarding higher risks of cardiovascular complications associated with their use, and some of them were removed from the market.

Thinning of the blood is another common side effect of some of the anti-inflammatory medications. This becomes an issue if you are considering having surgery. Most spine surgeons will recommend stopping all anti-inflammatory medications one or two weeks before surgery. That's because these medications can cause increased bleeding, which makes it much more difficult for your spine surgeon to operate. You may also find that you bruise easily, since your blood does not coagulate as efficiently when you are taking anti-inflammatory medications. The medication that is most commonly associated with thinning of the blood and decreasing the effectiveness of your platelet function is aspirin, the anti-inflammatory drug with which you are probably most familiar.

Rarer side effects of the NSAIDs include liver and kidney damage. Some patients who have taken massive doses of NSAIDs have suffered kidney failure. Some spine surgeons will also tell you to avoid these medications if you are having fusion surgery because NSAIDs can substantially slow down bone growth at the surgical site, which can lead to failure of the surgery. Because of these potential side effects, most doctors recommend that you do not take anti-inflammatory medications on a long-term basis. If you have been taking these medications for more than one month, your doctor may decide to do periodic blood work to check your liver and kidney functions.

Steroidal anti-inflammatory medications such as cortisone, dexamethasone, methylprednisolone, and Depo-Medrol are used much less frequently than nonsteroidal anti-inflammatory medications. This is because steroidal medications are much more potent than the NSAIDs and have many more side effects. They can cause more severe symptoms of gastritis and have other specific and potentially devastating side effects, such as stopping the blood flow to your hip joint. This is a rare complication, but it is still a possibility that must be considered when using this class of medication. For this reason, steroidal anti-inflammatory medications are usually given for only a few days to fight severe symptoms that are unbearable.

Muscle Relaxants

Muscle relaxants such as Valium, Robaxin, Fexeril, Skelaxin, and Soma can reduce muscle spasm and in turn reduce the pain that accompanies many spinal conditions. You may benefit from these medications and rest more comfortably, at least initially, when your symptoms are at their worst. Even though these medications are classified as muscle relaxants, their specific action for reducing pain is not entirely understood. It is hypothesized that they result in drowsiness, which in turn can relax your muscles.

This class of drug does not affect the cause of your problem, but only improves your pain while the medication is in your body. Still, muscle relaxants can be effective if you recently injured your back. Most injuries that result from lifting or abnormal movements are caused by muscle spasms and local inflammation. For this reason, muscle relaxants can be helpful in acute injuries, usually for only a few days after the injury has occurred. If your pain lasts more than a few weeks, muscle relaxants will be ineffective in providing you any long-lasting improvement. This is because most injuries and pain that last beyond a few weeks are not caused by muscle strain alone.

The various muscle relaxants have different potencies, potential for addiction, potential for causing drowsiness, and duration of action. Your doctor will choose the appropriate medication based on his own familiarity with the medication, his experience, and his knowledge of side effects and drug interactions.

Pain Medications

Pain medications such as Vicodin, Percocet, Vicoprofen, and Norco are also commonly prescribed for back pain. Most pain medications are derivatives of opiates and other narcotics, such as morphine and codeine. They directly fight chemicals that produce pain, and most have some addictive potential. There are two different components to addiction. One is tolerance and the other is dependency. Tolerance describes that fact that your body learns to process the medication more efficiently and, as a result, you may not feel the same beneficial effect after a few weeks or months of using it. For this reason, you may end up needing higher and higher doses to get the same pain-relieving effect. Dependency means that your brain gets used to having these medications and you can develop a drug-seeking behavior that is not in response to the pain.

There is a balance that must be maintained between pain relief and overuse of these medications. Your doctor can guide you in their appropriate use. In fact, there is a medical specialty dedicated to pain management. Doctors who specialize in pain management are usually anesthesiologists who have completed one year of specialized training in pain management. Your spine surgeon may refer you to such a doctor if your need for pain medication is complicated, or in cases where dependency and tolerance have developed.

As with other classes of medications, many different pain medications are available and each one is available in various dosages. Some are fast-acting, for severe, sudden pain; others are taken periodically, every few hours; and still others are available in the extended-release format and are used daily. Pain medication patches are also an option. Doctors try to prescribe the least amount of medication to control pain and maintain function. The stronger the medication and the longer you have taken these medications, the higher your chances of encountering complications.

Your physician will be guided by the information you have provided him. That's why it is so important to give your doctor accurate information. If you underestimate and describe your pain as mild, your doctor will attempt to use weaker medications to relieve your pain, which can result in undertreatment. If you overestimate your pain, however, and complain of severe, debilitating pain, stronger, more potent medications will be used. Keep in mind that you have the responsibility to convey accurate information so that appropriate medications are prescribed to you.

If your doctor attempts to decrease the strength of your medications, he is being conscientious and is practicing good medicine. Some pain management doctors place their patients on a strict schedule to avoid overutilizing these medications. They may even ask patients to sign a formal contract before they begin treating them. These contracts dictate the rules that are followed when using pain medications and the rules regarding medication refills and follow-up appointments.

Sleep Medications

Pain not only causes musculoskeletal dysfunction; it also has psychological consequences, such as depression, mood changes, and sleep disorders. Many patients who complain of pain have difficulty sleeping. Lack of sleep by itself can lead to an array of other consequences and increase your sensitivity to pain. Patients who get a good night's sleep can cope with pain much more effectively. Your doctor may consider prescribing sleep medications such as Dalmane, Restoril, or Ambien for a short period if you need them. Sleep medications do have addictive potential, however, and may cause more harm than good on a long-term basis. Your doctor can decide which medication is appropriate for you and how long you should use it.

Nerve-Stabilizing Medications

If you are suffering from nerve pain, which can be characterized by numbness, sharp discomfort, or abnormal sensation that radiates to your arms or legs, nerve-stabilizing medications can be of some help. The exact mechanism by which they reduce this type of pain is still unknown, but animal studies have shown that these medications reduce pain produced by nerve dysfunction. These medications are also used in patients who have diabetes-related nerve pain. Examples of such medications are Neurontin (gabapentin), Lyrica (pregabalin), and Elavil (amitriptyline). They are used for other disorders as well and should be used with caution. Neurontin is used to suppress seizures, but stopping the medication suddenly may actually result in a seizure. Elavil, on the other hand, is used to treat depression. Stopping it abruptly may result in depression and worsening of your pain. It is difficult to predict which of these medications will work best for you and, unfortunately, it often requires trial and error to find out.

Topical Medications

Topical medications can act locally or be absorbed through the skin and have the same effects throughout your body. Like pain medications, they can also be delivered by patches. Opioid pain patches are usually reserved for patients on high amounts of medications. An example of this type of delivery system is the Duragesic patch. It releases a constant flow of the opioid drug into the body and eliminates the ebbs and flows of the drug that occur when you take the medication orally. Other types of patches include one that delivers a numbing medication—lidocaine (also used by dentists)—locally to the area of pain. The most common of these types of patches is the Lidoderm patch. It can be applied once daily to the area of pain, but should be removed after twelve hours to avoid excessive delivery of the drug to your body. Even after you remove the patch, the effects of the medication will last for another twelve hours. If you are not allergic to the drug in the patch, you may derive benefit from using this medication for back and neck pain. A Lidoderm patch will not provide any benefit for nerve pain radiating to your arms or legs, since it only acts locally. Furthermore, these patches only treat the symptoms of your problem, not the cause. This patch is relatively safe, however, with very limited side effects.

Also available are various creams that can treat pain locally. Common over-the-counter creams include brands like Icy Hot, Bengay, and Capsin. These creams act locally and produce a sensation of heat and other stimuli that divert the sensation of pain from your brain. They can be effective for mild pain and have low rates of side effects.

OTHER NONINVASIVE THERAPIES

These modalities of treatment are the next step up the ladder after medications. For the most part, they do not have irreversible effects, and at least three of them (physical therapy, Pilates, and yoga) involve strengthening your muscles to provide better support for the other structures of your spine. Let's examine them now one at a time.

Physical Therapy

Physical therapy is the most common and least controversial treatment for back pain. What is physical therapy? It usually prescribes movements of your muscles and back in strategic ways to strengthen specific muscles, along with improving your posture and increasing the flexibility of your joints, tendons, and muscles. Most commonly, physical therapy is provided by a physical therapist, but chiropractors or other practitioners may also do it. Even though most back pain will resolve on its own, physical therapy can expedite your recovery and possibly also help you avoid recurrent episodes of back pain.

One of the basic concepts of physical therapy is to strengthen the back muscles so that they can provide more support for the other structures within the spine; stronger muscles can absorb the forces that affect the discs, joints, and ligaments of your spine. Endurance training is another important aspect of physical therapy. Your back muscles must provide continuous unrelenting support to your spinal column, while maintaining flexibility at the same time. No wonder that they tire, placing your spine at risk for injury. The longer your muscles can maintain their support, the less risk you will have for reinjury. This is called endurance. Flexibility is yet another key attribute that can be improved with therapy and exercise. The more flexible your muscles and tendons are, the more they can support and protect you in the different positions in which your spine may be placed.

Generally, women have problems that result from weak muscles, as compared with men, who have problems that are related to endurance. Most women will benefit from programs that strengthen their muscles and most men will benefit from programs that increase the endurance of muscle activity.

Physical therapists and other practitioners also offer additional treatments that include heat therapy, cold therapy, ultrasound, interferential muscle stimulation unit, massage therapy, acupressure (see page 46), reflexology, and cold laser. These passive modalities are generally used during the initial period after the injury to help you cope with the pain. Most of these therapies increase local blood flow or decrease inflammation. Generally, they do not have long-term benefits, and you can expect to see improvement of your symptoms for only a few hours.

Aquatherapy (water therapy) is another modality that uses the basic principles of physical therapy. Aquatherapy is performed in a pool, so that the water in effect reduces your weight, resulting in less stress to your joints when you perform exercises. You may feel protected in the water, which can have a psychological benefit, allowing you to perform more strenuous activities.

There are a few basic concepts that you should follow with every therapy program. You should always distinguish between deep, sharp pains as compared with muscle soreness, which may result from deconditioned muscles. You should also set a goal for your exercise program and should avoid going beyond that goal initially. As you start a physical therapy program, you may not feel that you have accomplished anything until a day later. At that time, you may feel intense muscle soreness that can actually slow you down. Because of that, most physical therapists will recommend that you start slowly and increase your level of activity over a few sessions. You should also avoid jerking movements or sudden extreme activity. Make your movements controlled and concentrate on the movement before you begin it.

Initially, perform a routine only for a few minutes. Increase that slowly over the next few sessions. If you begin an aerobic exercise, you may not be able to engage in it for more than two or three minutes at first. The next time, increase it to five or ten minutes, and then increase it to fifteen minutes. This can avoid any unnecessary frustration or the feeling that you cannot perform the exercise. This can also give you a sense of accomplishment once you have achieved your goal, at which time, with the blessing of your physical therapist, you may decide to surpass your goal altogether. Always remember, twisting is the enemy of your back and should be avoided in any type of exercise program unless it is slow and controlled.

Chiropractic Manipulation

The principle underlying chiropractic manipulation is that small misalignments of the spine can cause pain locally. Although their claims are not well accepted, some chiropractors argue that the key to other illnesses (including diabetes and childhood ear infections) lies in the spine, and that the correction of these misalignments can treat or even cure some medical conditions. Unfortunately, these misalignments often cannot be detected by X-ray unless they are severe, but they can be felt by a chiropractor. Practitioners of this therapy believe that manipulation of the spine moves the joints, tendons, and ligaments into their appropriate positions.

Chiropractic manipulation often produces a distinct sound and a sensation of relief, which is the hallmark of this type of therapy. The downside of chiropractic treatment is that the benefit only lasts a few hours and you may require long-term treatment to find lasting relief. There have been reports of catastrophic complications when patients with fractures or tumors have had chiropractic manipulation. Chiropractors undergo three or four years of training to reduce these risks as much as possible.

Acupuncture

Acupuncture is an age-old technique that relies on the placement of tiny needles in specific locations to reduce pain and dysfunction. These locations have been mapped by an ancient philosophy that is still used today. The exact mechanism by which acupuncture reduces pain is unknown and much controversy exists regarding its effectiveness for long-term pain relief. One theory is that the tiny needles placed in the skin redirect the pain signals and divert them away from the brain. Another theory suggests that the needles cause the release of endorphins (naturally produced morphine within your own body), which in turn reduces pain. Consider this to be like asking your own body to produce pain medication locally.

Acupressure uses a similar concept; focal pressure in specific areas can redirect pain signals and produce beneficial effects. There are no definitive scientific studies demonstrating the benefits of these treatments. They pose a low-risk option, however, and are at least worth a try.

Pilates and Yoga

The exercise techniques of Pilates and yoga, although they have been around for decades and centuries, respectively, have recently become popular and offer promising results to chronic back sufferers. They instruct participants in controlled movements of muscles that are not used during routine daily activities. These are called *core exercises* and promote the development of the muscles that are responsible for balance and posture. Yoga also uses powerful mental techniques and meditation for relaxation.

In moderation, these exercises can be helpful; extreme twisting and bending, however, can aggravate or even cause injury. As with any other exercise, start slowly and increase the intensity to a point that is comfortable for you. Some instructors may motivate you to reach above and beyond your goals, which may result in further injury.

The unique benefit of yoga is, as mentioned above, its use of meditation and mental relaxation. Otherwise, it uses the same basic principles of strengthening, stretching, and endurance training common to other types of exercise programs. Pilates also employs similar concepts but through the use of specialized equipment that utilizes the weight of your own body to produce resistance for muscle activity while avoiding significant movement. The exercises focus on muscle strengthening and endurance training while also emphasizing flexibility and stretching. Pilates uses all the principles of physical therapy with the added advantage of promoting weight loss. Pilates is not for you, however, if you have recently had a flare-up of back pain or have suffered a new back injury. Pilates and yoga should be used as a way of life when recovering from chronic back pain or in maintaining a healthy back.

PAIN MANAGEMENT PROCEDURES

Better understanding of the causes of back pain has led to the development of various modalities of pain management. Your pain management specialist has been trained in injection techniques and has knowledge of the most potent pain medications.

Epidural injections are one of the most common types of treatment offered by pain specialists. These are performed by placing a needle in a specific area of your spine and injecting steroid medications to combat inflammation. Other types of injections include facet blocks and discograms, which are performed either to diagnose or treat your condition. Most of these procedures are performed under X-ray visualization. Commonly, when performing one of these percutaneous procedures (i.e., through the skin), your spine specialist will use a *fluoroscopy unit*—a machine that allows him to take an X-ray picture and immediately see the image on a television screen. It also permits these X-ray pictures to be taken from various angles, which allows the physician to place a needle with great accuracy in almost any area of your body.

Epidural Injection

Epidural injections are performed by pain management specialists to treat back pain that radiates to your arm or leg. They are used to treat the pain caused by cervical, thoracic, and lumbar disc herniations, cervical spinal stenosis, and lumber spinal stenosis. You may have heard of epidural injections administered during childbirth. Epidural injections for back problems are somewhat different, since they are not meant to numb your extremities and there is no need to place a catheter in the spine. They simply deliver a small amount of steroid medication such as Celestone, cortisone, or Depo-Medrol locally around the nerves with a needle, which is removed immediately after the injection. If, for example, you are suffering from spinal stenosis or a disc herniation, your nerves are inflamed and swollen. Oral medication is distributed throughout your body and some of that medication is delivered through your blood to the area of inflammation. An epidural injection, by contrast, can deliver the medication with pinpoint accuracy to the area around the nerve, which results in much higher concentrations of the medication where it is needed most.

Most pain management specialists will perform epidural injections in an operating room under fluoroscopic guidance. Some specialists perform these injections in their office without the fluoroscopic imaging; the accuracy of the injections performed without fluoroscopic imaging, however, is usually lower. There are no specific recommendations in regard to the number of epidural injections that can be given or how often they should be administered. A general guideline is to perform a series of three injections, one week apart. This sequence usually insures adequate delivery of the medication to the affected area.

You can ask your doctor to make you drowsy before the injection so that you are very comfortable throughout the procedure. Expect to walk immediately afterward, with some soreness locally in the area of the injection. You may obtain benefit from the injection within one or two days. How long an injection will improve your symptoms is unpredictable. At best, the effects usually wear off after a few months. So, even though epidural injections have a relatively low rate of side effects, you should carefully consider your options because they don't work on all patients and their effects are usually temporary. Epidural injections have not been shown to change the final outcome if surgery is actually needed. The injections can, however, delay the need for surgery for a few months.

A common misconception is that epidural injections can weaken the bones in your body. This is generally not the case with epidural steroid injections, since the amount of medication is low and they are usually performed only a few times. By contrast, if you are using oral steroids to treat other conditions, such as lupus or rheumatoid arthritis, the medication can cause deterioration in bone density.

Selective Nerve Root Block

Selective nerve root blocks are usually regarded as a special type of epidural injection. The specialist administering a nerve root block injects cortisone, as in an epidural injection, as well as a numbing medication, around one single nerve into the neural foramen. Selective nerve root blocks can decrease pain if the area of concern is localized to one single nerve. Selective nerve root blocks can also be used as a diagnostic tool. If your spine surgeon has a question regarding the specific nerve that is under pressure, then selective nerve root block may provide the answers. For example, if your spine specialist suspects that a disc protrusion is placing pressure around the L4-5 neural foramen, a selective nerve root block at that level can confirm or contradict the diagnosis. This can be very helpful before surgery and may guide your spine surgeon to perform surgery on one specific disc level instead of multiple levels. In some cases, therefore, selective nerve root blocks can provide information that substantially increases surgical success rates.

Facet Block

Facet blocks are another common pain management procedure that can be used to diagnose or treat back pain. The facet joints, as we have seen, are the small joints in the rear of the spine that connect the vertebrae to one another. Just like any other joint in your body, they can develop pain and stiffness. Arthritis can cause the facet joints to enlarge and develop irregular surfaces, which can lead to pain when you attempt to move your spine. Inflammation of the sensory nerves attached to these joints can also cause pain. The location of these very small nerves is known and inflammation can be reduced by steroid medications delivered next to them. Facet blocks are performed in a manner similar to epidural injections, including the use of fluoroscopic guidance. Sometimes anesthetic medications are injected into the facet joints to see if your pain is originating from those joints. If you have immediate pain relief after an injection of an anesthetic medication in and around the facet, we can conclude that your pain is originating at least in part from the facet joint.

To you, a facet block will feel just like an epidural injection, since the only difference between the two is the location of the injection. In the operating room, you will probably be given sedatives before the facet block is performed. The skin is numbed and the needle is placed under fluoroscopic (X-ray) guidance. The needle is advanced to and around the facet joint. An injection, usually to the neck, mid-, or lower back, is performed, and then the needle is removed. An experienced pain management specialist can usually administer these injections in one or two minutes. Like epidural injections, they are performed in a series of two or three, a week apart. More than one joint can be injected at the same time if an MRI or CT scan has shown irregularity or enlargement of multiple facet joints.

Rhizotomy

If you have already had facet blocks performed and found obvious improvement in your symptoms, then rhizotomy may be the next logical step in treating your back pain. Rhizotomy destroys the small nerves that are located next to the facet joints and that transmit pain information from the facet joints to the brain. This procedure is performed in a manner similar to a facet block except that heat is applied for a few minutes with a small needle next to the nerve around the facet joint. Rhizotomy blocks the pathway for the sensation of pain that originates from the facet joints. The drawback of rhizotomy procedures is that the effect does not last forever. These nerves can regenerate and the pain may recur. Some spine specialists suggest repeating the rhizotomy procedure every six months to control your pain. The effects of repeated rhizotomy procedures may be longer-lasting than the first one.

Discogram

Discograms are often done purely as diagnostic tools. If you and your spinal specialist are in search of the cause of your back pain and for the specific disc that is causing it, then a discogram may be the next logical diagnostic test.

It is known that a normal disc will not produce pain when a needle is placed in it and fluid injected into it. By contrast, an abnormal disc *will* usually produce pain—and may reproduce the back pain you feel on a daily basis—when fluid is injected into it, increasing the pressure within the disc or irritating the tear if one is present. If you and your surgeon have decided to proceed with a surgical fusion of your spine, your surgeon may request a lumbar discogram prior to the surgery. This will provide information regarding the specific discs that are causing your back pain, thereby preventing your surgeon from fusing unnecessary disc levels. The goal is to perform the least invasive surgery while achieving the best surgical outcome, most improvement of symptoms, and the longest-lasting effect.

Discograms can be performed in the cervical or lumbar spine; in the cervical spine, however, they pose a much higher risk due to the difficulty of approaching the disc without causing injury to major vessels and nerves, the esophagus, the trachea, or the spinal cord. In the lumbar spine, the needles are placed obliquely to avoid injury to nerves and to the abdominal contents. Since in most cases, a discogram will be performed on the lumbar spine, I will describe a lumbar discogram.

Under the guidance of fluoroscopy, a needle is placed within each of three or four discs. Once all the needles are in the discs, fluoroscopy confirms their positions. A dye that increases the pressure within the disc is injected. Your doctor will then ask you two very important questions. One question is whether you feel pain when he is injecting the dye, and the second is about the quality of the pain. The presence of pain alone does not make a discogram positive. In order for a discogram to be positive, the test must reproduce the same type of pain that you feel every day. This is called a "concordant positive discogram." A painful disc that does not reproduce the same quality of pain is a negative discogram. The test will usually be performed over a few disc levels. Your doctor will want to test the reliability of the discogram by placing a needle and dye in a disc that appears normal, as well as a disc that appears abnormal. Your doctor would expect a pain-free disc if the MRI on that specific disc level is normal. In contrast, pain should be reproduced at the disc level that looks abnormal on the MRI.

Some doctors will obtain a CT scan after a discogram to examine the internal structure of the disc. More information can be obtained from a CT scan after a discogram has been performed. This is called a CT-discogram. A common finding on a CT-discogram is an annular tear, or a tear in the outer covering of the disc, which can cause pain. If there is a tear in the annulus of the disc, the dye that is injected within the disc during the discogram can be seen seeping out of the disc through the annular tear.

Even though many surgeons do use a discogram as a diagnostic tool, some spine specialists do not believe in the accuracy and reliability of this test. This controversy notwithstanding, the discogram is the only test that can prove that a disc is causing your back pain. As we have discussed, not all discs that look abnormal on an MRI will cause pain, and therein lies the value of a discogram. The discogram itself provides information regarding the severity as well as the character of the pain, and the CT scan provides the visual information regarding the integrity and shape of the disc.

Conversely, even if you have a positive discogram, your MRI study may show relatively normal images of your discs. This can pose a challenge to your spine surgeon in choosing the appropriate treatment plan for you. In most cases, if the puzzle does not fit, it's always safer to go the conservative route. In cases where the MRI is normal but the discogram reveals positive concordant pain, most spine specialists would suggest avoiding surgery and trying further conservative treatment to reduce pain and increase function.

Intradiscal Electrothermal Therapy (IDET)

In intradiscal electrothermal therapy (IDET) the outer envelope of the disc is heated and, in theory, a tear in the annulus is closed and the tiny nerves that transmit pain sensation from the disc to the brain are burned. Three or four years ago, this procedure was extremely popular for treating lower back pain and was regarded as a minimally invasive procedure with relatively low risk.

The procedure is done in the operating room under deep sedation. Without sedation and anesthesia, the procedure would be extremely painful and could not be tolerated. The approach is similar to that of a discogram in that a needle is placed within the disc space. After placement of the needle, its position is confirmed using fluoroscopy, and a wire is passed through the needle into the center of the disc. As the wire passes within the disc, it comes very close to the outer covering of the disc. The wire is then attached to a machine that heats it up, theoretically burning the small nerves around the annulus of the disc. Following this procedure, the patient is initially required to use a brace and then to do specifically recommended exercises.

When IDET was first introduced, the only research articles available were written by the physicians who developed the procedure. The initial success rates recorded by those physicians were approximately 80 percent. As more research articles were introduced into the scientific community, however, it was found that the success rates were lower than those initial reports had documented. A careful search for recent studies on IDET outcomes indicated that it does produce moderate improvement in back pain.

There are conditions that will prevent you from having an IDET procedure, such as a disc herniation or radiation of pain from your back to the leg. If you have leg pain, it may be due to a herniated disc that is placing pressure on the nerves that travel to your leg. In that case, it is not advisable to undergo an IDET procedure, since there is a risk that the wire that is advanced into the disc might enter the spinal canal itself.

The IDET procedure should only be performed after a discogram has revealed concordant pain. Furthermore, the best results have been seen in patients who have only one abnormal disc. The rate of success decreases if you have multiple discs that are abnormal. Since the failure of the IDET procedure does not prevent you from having a more aggressive treatment such a lumbar fusion, however, you may consider this procedure as another option to treat your back pain.

It is worth noting that some spine surgeons have abandoned IDET procedures altogether because they do not provide reliable or consistent outcomes. In the geographic area of my practice, most spine surgeons have stopped performing IDET, and I have not performed this procedure for the past few years.

*   *   *

If your pain resolves with the conservative modalities that we discussed in this chapter, bravo! That is a wonderful outcome. You have succeeded in achieving the goal of defeating your back pain. If your pain has not decreased, however, you may want to consider climbing the ladder to more aggressive treatment options. Next, we will explore those surgical options, investigating their benefits and risks.

4

Surgical Options

Making a decision about back surgery would be easy if it were a life-or-death issue. Fortunately, though, that is rarely the case. Back surgery is almost always an elective procedure and a lifestyle choice. Do you want to take the risks of surgery in order to reduce or eliminate pain and discomfort, or can you tolerate the discomfort to avoid the risks? These kinds of questions are precisely what often make the choice seem so confusing and overwhelming.

What also adds to the anxiety is the complicated wording often used to describe the procedures and the various parts of your spinal anatomy. Sometimes it may seem that your surgeon is speaking another language—and, in many ways, that's just what it is. It is the language of your spine. Laminectomy and laminoplasty? Lumbar microdiscectomy? Nucleoplasty? You need to be able to tune in and understand quickly. This is your chance to become fluent in the language of your back. In order to help you make your decisions, we'll take a look at the overall risks of back surgery, in addition to defining and describing all the major surgeries of the neck and back.

If you are reading about the surgical options, you have probably already had your diagnosis and have tried conservative options with your spinal specialist, but your pain or weakness has still not resolved. In most cases, your surgeon will offer you the options of proceeding with surgery or continuing with conservative treatment. There are only a few reasons that surgery would be strongly recommended. The main goal of most spinal surgery is to increase your quality of life. For this reason, you must seriously consider the risks versus the benefits before making a decision to proceed.

What may compound the difficulty of making a decision is that your spinal surgeon will only be able to give you an estimate of the chances of your success, based on her previous experience and the published clinical data from other surgeons in the country. Most spine surgeons will inform you about possible risks, both predictable and unpredictable, prior to the surgery. The chances of the surgery's success will depend on the accuracy of the diagnosis, the complexity of the procedure, and any other medical conditions that you may have.

Even though most patients who undergo spine surgery will benefit from it, not all will. If your spine surgeon is giving you a guarantee of success, it is a good time to be getting a second opinion! There are only two reasons for your spine surgeon to claim a success rate of 100 percent: either she does not perform enough of the procedures or she is embellishing her record.

RISKS TO CONSIDER

The overall risks of surgery must always be considered and compared to the benefits the surgery can offer you. You should, of course, also consider the severity of your condition and weigh it against the risks and benefits of surgery. The following are some of the more common risks of surgery.

Infection

Infection is a very common risk of almost any surgical procedure. Surgeries that require the placement of metallic implants in your body, as some spinal surgeries do, will inherently have a higher risk of infection. Between 3 percent and 7 percent of patients who receive metallic implants during surgery will suffer from this complication. The risk is much lower in patients who have surgery without metallic spinal implants. The reason for this is that bacteria hide from antibiotics and from the cells that fight infections within the crevices of the implants. In general, surgeries that use smaller incisions and that are performed faster have a lower risk of infection. The longer a wound is open, the longer bacteria have to get into the wound and cause an infection. In addition, during long procedures, the blood supply to the tissues is disrupted for a longer period of time, which can also increase the chances of infection.

There are other factors that contribute to the increased risk of infection. These include the defense mechanisms of your body. If you have diabetes or any disease that affects your immune system, such as HIV infection or AIDS, your chances of infection are much higher. Some medications that reduce your immune response, such as steroids, also increase the risk. If you develop an infection after an operation, the treatment options could be as simple as taking medications for seven days or as complicated as requiring multiple additional surgeries. These could include the removal of any metallic implants that your surgeon placed in your spine during the original surgery. In order to avoid infection, most surgeons routinely provide patients with antibiotics prior to the surgery. In surgical procedures in which metallic implants are used, your surgeon may consider administering antibiotics after the surgery as well.

Dural Tear

As we have seen, the dura is the tough envelope and outer covering that surrounds the spinal cord and the brain, which are bathed in a fluid called the cerebrospinal fluid (CSF). The body makes about 240 cc (cubic centimeters) of CSF every day. As this fluid is produced and delivered into the dural sac, the same amount of CSF is reabsorbed into the bloodstream and removed from the dural sac. Thus, the amount of CSF around your brain and spinal cord remains constant.

Dural tears can occur during a variety of procedures, including pain management procedures such as discograms and epidural injections. Dural tears occur much more frequently in revision surgery due to the significant scar tissue that develops around the spine from the first surgery.

If there is an inadvertent tear of the dura, the CSF will begin to leak from the dural sac into the surgical wound. In most cases, there will be continuous drainage of clear fluid from the wound and this will be easily detectable by your surgeon. If possible, your surgeon will suture the tear to attain watertight closure. There are many different techniques used to close dural tears, but all have the same goal: to achieve a watertight closure to stop any leakage into the wound.

Since there is supposed to be a specific amount of fluid within the dural sac, which also surrounds the brain, a leakage can result in severe headaches. This type of pain can worsen if you stand or walk. The reason for the increase in pain is that when you walk, more fluid comes out of the tear due to gravity. In a standing position, the amount of fluid around your brain decreases even more, worsening the severity of the headaches.

Dural tears that occur inadvertently during pain management procedures are usually very small and in most cases resolve spontaneously at some point. Uncommonly, they do not heal and require the injection of blood into the area of the tear to act as glue so that the tear will close up. This procedure is called a *blood patch* and is usually effective in treating these small dural tears.

Occasionally, the CSF may continue to leak until another surgery is performed to repair the tear. Not all tears, however, can be repaired during surgery. If the tear is not accessible to your surgeon, she can place special glue over it, along with local muscle tissue, to close the tear until your own body heals it on its own.

If you have suffered from a dural tear that was not seen during surgery, your best option is to lie flat in bed for a few days and drink tea that has high levels of theophyline in it. Theophyline is known to increase production of CSF, which will decrease your headaches until the tear can heal by itself. If the tear has been repaired, most spine surgeons also recommend bed rest for about three days. This will reduce the pressure of CSF over the repair site; the less pressure placed on the site of repair, the faster the tear will heal. Some surgeons place a catheter within the dural sac to drain out the CSF. This reduces the pressure on the repaired dura, allowing it to heal faster. If a tear in the dura occurs during the surgery and goes undetected, the leaking CSF can result in a cyst that fills with this fluid. If the cyst closes, it will act as an outpouching of the dural sac, and in most cases, will not have long-term consequences.

Pseudarthrosis

Pseudarthrosis is a complication that can occur if you have undergone a procedure to fuse a segment of your spine. The concept behind fusion surgery is to stop a segment of the spine from moving. This is usually performed by removing a disc and placing bone in the area that was previously mobile. The added bone welds and fuses the two surrounding vertebrae. If this attempt at bony fusion is not successful, you will still have movement in that segment of the spine, which may or may not become painful. If the failure of the bones to fuse is detected on an X-ray or a CT scan, it is called a pseudarthrosis. It's not always an easy diagnosis to make, however. In some cases, it is difficult to see the problem on an X-ray and it may even be difficult to detect on a CT scan. The best way to check for pseudarthrosis is to reopen the incision surgically and look at the fusion site.

Much effort has been put into research to increase chances of fusion and reduce the risk of pseudarthrosis. In fact, one of the main purposes of metallic implants is to reduce the risk of this complication. If you are undergoing a fusion procedure, your spine surgeon may consider inserting metallic implants to stop any movement until the bone fuses. After the fusion has occurred, usually in about three to five months, the metallic implants will no longer have any function. On the other hand, if the fusion does not take place, the metallic implants will have to bear most of the burden in preventing movement in that segment of the spine. Eventually, complications can occur, since metallic implants are not designed to immobilize your spine indefinitely. They can break or loosen and cause further pain.

Even if you have been diagnosed with pseudarthrosis, however, you may not necessarily have pain. Many patients with pseudarthrosis will have no pain at all. If you do have pseudarthrosis after spine surgery and you require more treatment to relieve residual pain, you should choose your spine surgeon very carefully, making sure that she is experienced in treating patients who have failed initial surgery on their spine. Revision surgery is much more complicated than the first one and usually has a lower rate of success.

Neurological Injury

During surgical procedures on the spine, you are at risk of suffering further injury to your nerves. Neurological injury can range from vague numbness in a small area like the foot to catastrophic paralysis after surgery. In different regions of the spine, there are different risks. A major anatomical consideration is that the spinal cord ends at the upper part of the lower back—at the L1 or L2 vertebral body level. Therefore, while the spinal cord is at risk with surgeries to the cervical, thoracic, and upper lumbar spines, the risk of paralysis is much less with surgery on the lower lumbar spine.

Surgeries that are performed to relieve conditions of the neck place the spinal cord at greatest risk and can cause complete paralysis at and below the level of surgery. Fortunately, this complication is rare; the risk of paralysis from surgery to the cervical spine is less than 1 percent in most cases. This is because it is of utmost concern to any spine surgeon to protect the spinal cord during surgery.

In the lumbar spine, damage to specific nerves is more common than damage to the spinal cord. Below the L1 or L2 vertebra, where the spinal cord ends, many nerves descend and exit the spine through multiple exit holes called the neural foramina. Each nerve has a specific function and causes different symptoms when damaged. Injury to the nerves can result from the pulling of a nerve, also called a traction injury. Traction of nerves is commonly required to remove a herniated disc or to place a metallic implant. Inadvertent laceration of a nerve is a much more serious complication that can also result in numbness, weakness, and pain. Placement of pedicle screws can also increase the risk of nerve injury. If the screw is misplaced, it can place pressure on a nerve and can lead to nerve dysfunction after the surgery. The best way to detect a badly positioned pedicle screw is with a CT scan.

Surgical approaches to the spine through the abdomen pose lower risk to the nervous structures because they allow your spine surgeon to visualize, and have excellent access to, the large vertebral body. The anterior approach, however, encounters major blood vessels, and injury to those vessels can cause rapid bleeding. Approaches through the rear of the spine, on the other hand, involve increased risk of injury to the nerves because of their location, closer to the back of the spine.

Nerve injury can also result from other causes, such as bleeding within the spinal canal after the surgery. Often, however, the reason for neurological injury remains unknown. In many cases, a neurological deficit will improve on its own within a few days. Some surgeons will recommend using cortisone-based medications to reduce inflammation, which increases the chances of neurological recovery.

Medical and Anesthetic Complications

The risk of medical and anesthetic complications depends on your prior medical history, as well as your specific age group. If you suffer from diabetes or have had a heart attack, you will be at a higher risk of complications, and anticipating those possibilities can reduce the chances that they will occur. Some possible complications are strokes, blood clots in your legs, and anesthetic problems. There have been multiple research studies showing the risk of anesthesia—the risk of death is estimated at 1 in 700,000—but it is very difficult to demonstrate the exact risk for each different potential complication. In most cases, your spine surgeon will request a preoperative medical clearance from a cardiologist or an internist to minimize the risk of medical complications.

TYPES OF SURGERY

Once you have weighed the reasons for surgery, and if—like millions of others in pain—you decide to proceed with it, you should become familiar with each type of surgery, as well as the risks that accompany it. In general, two types of surgeries can be performed on your spine. The first is decompression and the other is fusion. Depending upon your problem, they can be performed separately or as a combined procedure.

A decompressive procedure is one that attempts to remove the pressure on the nervous structures, which may include individual nerve roots or the spinal cord itself. The pressure can result from a protruding disc, an enlarged facet joint, tumors, deformity, or a cyst protruding from a facet joint, also called a *synovial cyst*. Laminectomy, laminotomy, microdiscectomy, foraminotomy, laminoplasty, discectomy, microendoscopic discectomy, endoscopic discectomy, and laser discectomy are examples of this type of procedure. A decompression procedure is performed to improve the symptoms you have in your arms or legs and will usually not improve lower back or neck pain. This is the reason your surgeon will keep asking you the location of your pain and comparing the pain in your back with that in your arms or legs.

As mentioned previously, an operation called a fusion attempts to stop any movement in a specific segment of your spine. By preventing movement in an abnormal segment of the spine, we hope that the pain originating from that area will stop as well. Multiple problems in your spine can cause pain, as we have seen, including arthritis, deformity, cancer, or repeated disc herniation. Degenerative disc disease and arthritis are common causes of back pain, which may or may not be associated with pain in the arms or the legs. In most cases, a decompression procedure will not improve this kind of axial (mechanical) back pain. Fusion procedures, although imperfect, are performed to reduce axial back pain. Generally, fusion operations are much more technically demanding and take longer than decompression procedures.

Other procedures have been introduced in recent years that differ from decompression and fusion surgery. Kyphoplasty and vertebroplasty, for instance, are procedures that reduce the pain of specific types of fractures, and these procedures cannot be categorized as decompression or fusion surgeries.

Decompression Surgery

The goal of all surgeries that decompress spinal nerves and the spinal cord is to reduce pain and dysfunction resulting from pressure on the nerves. This type of surgery can be performed alone, or in combination with fusion surgery. In most cases, decompressive surgery is simpler and faster to perform than fusion surgery. Examples of this type of surgery include the well-known microdiscectomy and laminectomy. During surgery, your doctor will remove some bone, as well as ligaments, to approach the nerves or the spinal cord. At that time, a herniated disc, or any other tissue that is compressing the neural elements, can be removed. The more bone that your surgeon removes during surgery, the more risk you have of developing a deformity and abnormal motion between segments of your spine later on in life. There is a delicate balance between removing enough bone to alleviate the pressure on your nerves and keeping enough bone within the facet joints to avoid development of instability. In cases where too much bone was removed to decompress the nerves, your surgeon may decide to fuse that segment of the spine in order to avoid the onset of instability and deformity later on.

Fusion Surgery

Let's take a more detailed look at fusion surgery. As I mentioned, fusing segments of the spine is a very common surgical option in treating spinal conditions. Many of the problems that we encounter within our spine are caused by movement in a specific segment resulting in degeneration, which, in turn, can cause disc herniations, instability, and other common conditions. Surgically fusing a segment is similar to welding two parts of bone to each other. In attempting to fuse bones, we actually try to make bone grow in places it did not exist before—that is, in an area from which we have removed a disc, inside a facet joint, or between transverse processes. To do this, we must help the body create new bone. This can be accomplished by bringing bone from other parts of the body or by using chemicals that are known to stimulate bone growth.

The act of transferring bone is called *bone grafting*. Bone grafting is the most common way to fuse bones to each other. If a bone graft is obtained from other body parts within the same person—most commonly, the pelvis—it is called *auto-grafting*. If bone is obtained from another person, it is called *allo-grafting*. Auto-grafting has the best potential for stimulating bone growth, since it includes active, live cells as well as structural bone. In contrast, an allo-graft usually includes only the framework of the bone, without any live cells. Recently, the chemical that is naturally produced in our bodies to stimulate bone growth was synthetically produced and introduced to the market. This chemical is called bone morphogenetic protein (BMP), and it is frequently used by spine surgeons to enhance the success rates of their surgery.

In order to increase the chances of a fusion, surgeons commonly use metallic implants to immobilize the segment of the spine that is to be fused. The most common type of metal used for implantation is titanium. Previously, stainless steel was used, but titanium is used more commonly today because of its implant compatibility with MRI and other diagnostic technology. Pedicle screws are the most common implants used in the lumbar spine, and metallic screws with plates are most common in the cervical spine. Many other types of implants are available, but the basic concept behind most of the implants is the same; they are to be attached to the bone to prevent movement in that segment of the spine. The exception to this rule is the newer treatment of disc replacement, which I will describe later in this chapter.

Surgeries of the Cervical Spine (Neck)

We have covered the basic issues involved in decompressive and fusion surgery. Next we will discuss the specific surgeries that are used to treat the conditions of your neck.

Anterior Cervical Discectomy and Fusion (ACDF)

Anterior cervical discectomy and fusion is one of the most common procedures performed in the neck. The term *anterior* simply means that the neck is approached from the front. The term *cervical* refers to the neck, and the term *discectomy* simply means removal of the disc to decompress the spinal cord and the nerves.

If you are suffering from a disc herniation, cervical myelopathy, cervical instability, or discitis (infection of the disc), your spine surgeon may offer you this procedure. Of course, you should already have attempted appropriate nonsurgical options before resorting to surgery. If you are considering this type of surgery, however, there is some good news. This is the second most common procedure performed by spine surgeons and it is generally agreed that it is usually very successful in achieving a good outcome. In addition, the pain associated with ACDF is relatively low compared with other types of spine surgery.

Let's take a look at how the surgery is performed. After you are completely anesthetized, your spine surgeon will make an incision approximately three inches long in the front, left side of your neck. If the operation is performed on one or two levels, most surgeons will choose to place a horizontal incision in line with the skin creases. This makes the incision more cosmetically pleasing. Surgeons will usually choose to use a vertical incision if the surgery is going to be performed on three or four levels. In most cases, the incision heals nicely and the scar is difficult to see a year later.

After penetrating the skin, the surgeon encounters a thin layer of muscle, which is incised along the lines of the skin incision. Going a bit deeper, the surgeon pushes a few larger vessels to the side. These vessels run alongside the trachea, or the windpipe, as well as the esophagus, which is the tube that takes food down into your stomach. The approach to the spine is made by spreading and going between the structures of the neck without cutting through them. This may be one reason that this type of surgery is usually not too painful.

During surgery, it is very important for the surgeon to make certain that the correct disc is being removed. This is usually achieved by taking an X-ray during the operation. The disc is then taken out, using special instruments. After removing the disc, the surgeon also cuts away small osteophytes (arthritic bony projections) from the neural foramen. This further releases any pressure from the nerves that exit the spine. Once the disc is removed, your surgeon has to fill the empty space from which the disc was taken. She accomplishes this by using a metallic implant, bone from the bone bank, or bone removed from your own pelvis.

Your spine surgeon has many options and she will chose the implant that is best for you. Using bone from your pelvis results in higher fusion rates, but 30 percent of patients who have bone removed from their pelvis will have some type of complication. For that reason, some surgeons will use donated bone from cadaveric sources. After placement of bone or a synthetic spacer within the disc space, your spine surgeon may choose to place a metallic implant in front of the spine to increase the rigidity of that specific segment, which also results in higher fusion rates. The metallic implant, however, can also cause complications; it can break and the screws can back out, which can cause difficulty with swallowing and a variety of other problems. In general, though, most spine surgeons do use a metallic implant when performing this type of surgery.

As with any surgery, ACDF carries its own risks and benefits beyond the general surgical ones we've already discussed. Infection is less common with surgery to the cervical spine, since there is good blood flow to the area. Pseudarthrosis (see page 58) occurs in 10 percent of patients, but only 30 percent of patients with pseudarthrosis will have residual pain. The risk of neurological injury is approximately 1 percent. A very uncommon complication is injury to the esophagus. Some patients may have difficulty swallowing. If you experience this problem, try to eat soft foods and gradually move to more solid foods. Difficulties eating usually resolve within six months. If your symptoms don't improve, you may require a second surgery to remove the metallic plates that were inserted in the original operation.

Another uncommon complication is damage to the recurrent laryngeal nerve, a small nerve that transmits the signal from your brain to your vocal cords in order to move them and produce sound. If the nerve is injured during the operation, one of your vocal cords will not work properly and you can have changes to your voice. In most cases, however, the nerve will recover and your voice will normalize as time passes. The anatomy of this nerve is more predictable on the left side, which is the reason most spine surgeons perform this surgery from the left side of the neck.

Posterior Cervical Foraminotomy

If you are suffering from a disc herniation in your neck that is pushing on a nerve in the neural foramen, you may have the option of undergoing a posterior cervical foraminotomy. As always, you should have attempted to resolve your problem using conservative treatment initially. In cases in which a single disc herniation is placing pressure on a nerve, the spine can be approached from the rear (posterior) instead of the front (anterior). Posterior foraminotomy surgery is not as commonly performed as anterior cervical discectomy and fusion. This is because the anterior approach often has excellent results, and there is much more muscle tissue that needs to be penetrated to gain access to the cervical spine from the rear. Posterior foraminotomy does not require a fusion as anterior cervical discectomy does. This operation only decompresses and relieves the nerves from the pressure that is being placed upon them by the disc.

So, then, why might you choose this surgery? The results of posterior foraminotomy surgery are somewhat less predicable, but it sidesteps some of the complications that can occur with anterior surgery. If you are a singer or you rely on your voice for work, most spine surgeons would suggest performing the surgery through the posterior approach, since there is no risk to your voice. The danger of damage to the esophagus and swallowing difficulties are also eliminated.

Let's take a look at how this surgery is performed. After you are completely anesthetized, in most instances, you are placed lying on your abdomen. A small incision is made vertically in the rear of your neck.

The muscles are then moved to the side, exposing the bone. A small hole is made in the bone, exposing the nerve. In most cases, the removal of the bone itself can decompress the nerve. The nerve can also be moved aside and the disc herniation removed. With a posterior foraminotomy, there is no need to fuse that level and the operation is complete once the nerve is decompressed. One of the risks of posterior foraminotomy, however, is cervical instability, which may create the need for a fusion anteriorly. In addition, if this surgery is performed in higher segments of the spine, the vertebral arteries can be placed at risk, which increases the chances of a stroke.

Cervical Laminectomy

If you are suffering from spinal stenosis (see page 26), in which there is pressure on your spinal cord and your nerves over multiple levels, you may require a laminectomy or a laminoplasty procedure. Cervical laminectomy refers to the removal of the lamina, which, as we saw earlier, is considered to be the roof of your spinal canal. The removal of the lamina creates more room for the nerves and the spinal cord, which can reduce or eliminate symptoms of arm pain and numbness, weakness, clumsiness in the hands, or difficulty walking. However, the removal of the lamina may also cause your spinal column to become unstable, and you may require further surgery in the form of a fusion. Fortunately, this is not common and will depend on the extent of the bone that has been removed during the original surgery.

As in a posterior foraminotomy, you will be placed on your stomach. An incision is made vertically over the center of your spine and the muscles are spread to the sides. Once the bone is fully exposed, a high-speed drill is used to remove the lamina. Very careful dissection is performed to avoid any injury to the spinal cord or the nerves that exit from the spinal column. In order to avoid instability after a laminectomy, some surgeons will choose to fuse the spine during the initial operation. This can be performed using metallic implants or by placing bone grafts along the sides of the remaining bone in the posterior aspect of the cervical spine. If screws and metallic implants are used, it is called "fusion with instrumentation"; if no metallic implants are used, your spine surgeon will call this "fusion without instrumentation." If the operation is performed without fusion, most spine surgeons will let you move your neck after the operation. If fusion is performed along with the laminectomy, however, you will be placed in a rigid cervical collar.

Cervical Laminoplasty

The term *laminoplasty* refers to a procedure that modifies the shape of the lamina. Instead of removing it completely, the surgeon creates an opening in the lamina and that piece of bone is elevated upward and away from the spinal cord and the nerves. This creates more room for the spinal cord and the nerves, achieving the same result as the laminectomy does. Research has shown that laminoplasty results in lower rates of instability later on. Most spine surgeons will not perform a fusion with a laminoplasty, but some research studies have shown an improved outcome when the surgery is performed with a cervical fusion. Research has also shown that laminoplasty creates more pain on a long-term basis. Controversy exists as to the best type of surgery, and the choice remains with you and your surgeon.

Posterior Cervical Fusion

You may need a cervical fusion if you are suffering from instability in your spine (i.e., abnormal movement in one segment of your spine), or if you had another surgery that resulted in the need for a fusion. If you are the unfortunate victim of a fracture that resulted in instability, you may need a fusion to the fractured segment. Some fractures can be treated by simple bracing, but not all will heal correctly.

As I have mentioned, bone to be used in the fusion can be obtained from your pelvis or from local bone that has been removed during a laminectomy procedure. A higher chance of fusion is obtained when screws and rods are used. The screws that are used in a posterior cervical fusion are called *lateral mass screws*. They are relatively small and must be precisely placed to avoid risk of injury to important structures of your neck. If you require a fusion, your spine surgeon will most likely place you in a brace for approximately three months after the surgery. This is because lateral mass screws are not as strong as screws that are inserted in other places in the spine.

Injury to the vertebral artery, which provides circulation to specific parts of your brain, is a danger when lateral mass screws are placed.

Injury to that artery can sometimes lead to strokes, but, fortunately, humans have arteries on both sides of the spine, which can compensate for injury to one side. As with any other fusion procedure, you will always face the risk of pseudarthrosis. If you have pain resulting from pseudarthrosis, you may need another surgery to graft more bone and possibly to change the screws that were placed in the original surgery.

Cervical Disc Replacement

If you required a cervical fusion previously, you may be part of the very small group of patients who will face degeneration and herniation of an adjacent disc level. The exact percentage of patients who suffer from adjacent level disc degeneration is still unknown, though the rate has been estimated to be anywhere from 1 to 10 percent. Adjacent level disc degeneration is hypothesized to occur because the fusion procedure places further stress on the adjacent levels and causes them to degenerate more rapidly. In order to avoid adjacent level degeneration, while still obtaining the benefits of removal of the abnormal disc, cervical disc replacement has been proposed. In Europe, the procedure is commonly performed, and in the United States it has recently been approved by the Food and Drug Administration. Lumbar disc replacement was approved recently, prior to the approval of cervical disc replacement. The benefits of a cervical disc replacement over a cervical fusion have been questioned by many spine surgeons, since we know that a cervical fusion has excellent outcomes and is a relatively simple procedure. The benefits of a cervical disc replacement, as opposed to a cervical fusion, will have to be examined in about ten years, after it has been widely performed. There is no doubt, however, that the companies that produce these implants will widely and aggressively market the procedure.

Surgeries of the Lumbar Spine

Lumbar spine (lower back) surgery is much more common than surgery of the cervical spine, since disorders of the lumbar spine are much more common than those of the neck. Even though the risk of paralysis is much less in the lumbar spine, risks of other complications are higher. This is because more of the body weight is distributed to the lower part of your spine and more physical demands are made of the lumbar spine compared with the cervical spine.

Lumbar Decompressive Procedures

Your spine surgeon will suggest a decompression if you are suffering from symptoms of numbness, weakness, or pain in your legs. Difficulty walking for more than a few minutes is another common problem that you may have if there is pressure on the nerves that exit from your spinal column. *Cauda equina syndrome* is the most severe condition that requires a decompression. As we saw in Chapter 1, the cauda equina is the collection of nerves that is located at the bottom of the spinal cord; it allows you to control urination and defecation. Pressure on these nerves can cause severe numbness and weakness in the legs, numbness around the genitals and the anus, and loss of bowel and bladder control. If left untreated, the loss of bladder and bowel control can become permanent and severely disabling. Cauda equina syndrome must be treated with emergency surgical laminectomy to remove the cause of pressure on the nerves. The best results are seen when decompression surgery is performed within twenty-four hours of the onset of symptoms.

As we've discussed, a decompression procedure simply removes pressure from the nerves in your lower back. An array of procedures is available, starting from a traditional multilevel open laminectomy to smaller types of operations such as discectomy, microdiscectomy, minimally invasive microdiscectomy, microendoscopic discectomy, endoscopic discectomy, and laser discectomy.

Lumbar Laminectomy. The removal of a section of the lamina (the "roof" of the spinal canal) is sometimes required and is called laminectomy, as we saw with regard to the cervical spine. If you are suffering from spinal stenosis and your symptoms have not resolved with conservative treatment, your spine surgeon will probably suggest a lumbar decompression.

Reviewing the anatomy will make it easier for you to understand the surgery. Each nerve exits the spinal column below the facet joint, through the neural foramen. In a lumbar laminectomy, the lamina is removed, along with the inner part of the facet joint, which is usually enlarged as a result of degenerative arthritis. In the world of spine surgery, this is called *medial facetectomy.* If the inner aspect of the enlarged facet joint is not removed along with the lamina, the nerve can remain under pressure and your symptoms may not resolve, even after surgery.

If too much of the facet joint is removed, that segment of your spinal column may become unstable and you may require a fusion surgery later on in life. So there is a delicate balance between removing too much bone, which results in instability of your spinal column, and keeping too much bone and not relieving the pressure on the nerves.

Laminectomy is a traditional, time-proven procedure and is the standard operation with which other procedures are compared. Results are generally good and you should expect relief from leg discomfort, cramping, and difficulty walking. It can take months before you will feel improvement in numbness, which usually depends upon the recovery of the nerve itself.

Another reason a laminectomy is performed is to treat an infection within the spinal canal. An infection can cause the collection of fluid, also called an abscess, within the spinal canal, which can place pressure on the nerves and the spinal cord itself. This condition is dangerous and can be life-threatening. In most cases, it requires surgery to remove the fluid and relieve the pressure. A laminectomy can efficiently accomplish this task.

To undergo a lumbar laminectomy, you will be completely anesthetized. The surgery is performed while you are lying on your abdomen on a special table—usually an Andrews table or a Wilson frame. An incision is made in the lower back across the levels of the spine that require the decompression. The muscles around the spinal column are dissected and moved to the side until the bone is exposed. The bone is removed, using a variety of instruments, which includes a high-speed drill. Some surgeons will use an operating microscope, while others use magnifying glasses. Proponents of the microscope argue that they can see much more detail. The magnifying glasses, however, allow the surgeon much more control and movement during surgery. Research studies also show lower rates of infection when magnifying glasses are used, since the relatively large microscope is not in the surgical field, eliminating the potential delivery of bacteria into the area.

Lumbar Microdiscectomy and Laminotomy. A microdiscectomy means excision of a disc using a microscope or a magnifying glass. Laminotomy means making a hole in the lamina. The microdiscectomy and laminotomy are performed through a smaller incision and require the removal of less bone than the laminectomy. If you are suffering from a disc herniation that is placing pressure on one specific nerve and you have tried conservative treatment that failed, then your answer may lie with this type of procedure. Of course, the specific nerve and level needing treatment must be diagnosed with an MRI prior to the surgery, so that the procedure can be directed to the appropriate disc level.

As with any other spine surgery, you are first fully anesthetized by the anesthesiologist. Then, you are placed on your abdomen and the surgeon is guided to the site of the incision by an X-ray image. Confirming the site of the incision with an X-ray assures you of having the smallest incision possible. If your anatomy is typical (and that is not always the case!) a very skilled surgeon can usually perform the surgery through a one-inch incision, but the average size is two to three inches. A smaller incision produces less postoperative pain and can mean a faster recovery. The risk of infection and bleeding is lower as well.

After making the incision, your surgeon will push aside the muscles to expose the lamina, using one of the many retractors available for this purpose. A small hole is made within the lamina (laminotomy). This will expose the ligamentum flavum, which is also called the yellow ligament. The spinal nerves are below this ligament. Once the ligament is removed, the nerve and the dura can be seen within the spinal canal. When a disc within your spine herniates, it places pressure on your spinal nerve from the bottom. The herniated disc then pushes the nerve back and crushes it against the ligamentum flavum and the lamina. The removal of the lamina and the ligamentum flavum will relieve a lot of pressure from the nerve. If your spine surgeon uses a nerve-monitoring computer, also called somatosensory evoked potential (SSEP), it will show improvement in the nerve function as soon as the ligament and the bone are removed.

After removal of a small piece of the bone and the ligament, the nerve can be visualized. By moving the nerve to the side, the herniated disc can be removed from the spinal canal and this is called a discectomy. The overgrowth of bone from arthritis can also place pressure on the exiting nerve. Facet arthritis and facet enlargement are very common and make the neural foramen very tight. The excision of this bony overgrowth and the enlargement of the neural foramen are called a *foraminotomy*.

In recent years, the advantages of smaller incisions and minimally invasive techniques have been appreciated by most spine surgeons and their benefits documented by multiple studies. As we have seen, the incision for a lumbar microdiscectomy is usually about two or three inches in length. The pain from the surgery usually comes from the incision and the dissection of the muscle in your back. In order to avoid this dissection and to perform the surgery through a smaller incision, minimally invasive procedures have been introduced, and I will discuss them next.

Microendoscopic Discectomy and Minimally Invasive Microdiscectomy. The concept behind a microendoscopic discectomy is the same as a microdiscectomy procedure. In fact, the only difference between these surgical techniques is the size of the incision. Surgeons who are trained to perform this surgery can also do the procedure faster, since the time for dissection is reduced. Not all spine surgeons are familiar with these more technically challenging procedures, but the move toward minimally invasive techniques and the increased demand from patients has forced many older-generation spine surgeons to learn and practice these procedures.

In the microendoscopic discectomy, an incision is made over the specific disc level that is herniated and a small tube is placed over the bone. A very small camera is then placed within the tube and a video picture is projected onto a television screen in the room. Your spine surgeon can look at the screen and perform the operation through the small tube. This has resulted in smaller incisions with less muscle dissection. A skilled surgeon can perform the operation through a one-inch incision. Since the incision is so small, there is less pain and patients can leave the surgery center or hospital the same day. After introduction of the microendoscopic discectomy, most spine surgeons noted that they could perform the procedure simply by using the microscope or special magnifying glasses through the same small tube. That introduced us to the minimally invasive microdiscectomy procedure. With this new technique, the video camera has almost become extinct and the use of magnifying glasses has become much more common.

As the technology for minimally invasive procedures has improved, spine surgeons have also become more comfortable performing these operations. One of the manufacturing companies introduced a set of instruments called the METRx instrument system, which allows spine surgeons to perform the microdiscectomy procedure with a one-inch incision using the tubes that I mentioned. As in the traditional microdiscectomy procedure, the appropriate disc level is identified and a small incision is made over it. Small dilators are placed within the incision up to the bone. The rest of the procedure is performed in the traditional fashion by making a small hole in the bone and exposing the ligamentum flavum, as well as the nerve. From then on, the herniated disc fragment can be removed and, if necessary, a foraminotomy can also be accomplished.

The advantage of this procedure is the very small incision and the fact that the muscles in your back are not damaged as much during the approach to the bone and the disc. Theoretically, your muscles are moved only slightly during the surgery, but, in reality, there is some muscle damage during any surgery! The extent of the muscle damage is lessened, however, using these minimally invasive procedures. If your spine surgeon is comfortable with this type of surgery, it can be performed in the same length of time or even less than the traditional type of surgery. Since a smaller incision is used with the minimally invasive approach, the risk of infection is also lower. With the minimally invasive approach, you should expect less pain than with the traditional surgery, and the recovery time is approximately one to two months. Recovery time with the traditional microdiscectomy procedure may be slightly longer because of the more extensive muscle damage.

Laser Discectomy, Percutaneous Discectomy, Nucleoplasty, and Endoscopic Discectomy. Over the past few years, many new surgical options have been introduced. Some spine surgeons have reported excellent and consistent success rates with these procedures. They have not been reproduced by other spine surgeons, however, and, for this reason, these procedures are not regarded as mainstream treatments for a disc herniation and—wisely—are not widely used.

Laser discectomy is a procedure by which a probe is introduced into the disc space. The laser ray burns a segment of the disc, which theoretically removes the disc material that pushes on the nerve. The problem with this procedure is that the laser beam cannot be adequately directed to the correct area. Long-term results have not confirmed the claims made by the few people who perform this procedure.

Percutaneous discectomy is a procedure in which a small probe is introduced into the disc space and a small shaver removes disc material from that area. Again, this is not a controlled procedure and has not produced consistent results. For this reason, it has been abandoned by most spine surgeons.

Nucleoplasty has been backed by a large marketing campaign and is mostly performed by anesthesiologists who have gone through a fellowship program in pain management. Mixed results have been observed with this procedure, but, again, long-term results have not been substantiated. The procedure involves placing a small tube that acts as a shaver in the disc space. This tube is connected to suction, which sucks out the disc material that the shaver removes.

Endoscopic discectomy is a procedure in which a large volume of disc material is removed using special instruments. First, a needle is introduced into the disc and then a blue dye is injected into it. The theory behind this procedure is that only abnormal disc material will absorb the blue dye. A very small camera is then placed into the disc space. While the disc space is visualized, any disc material that has absorbed the dye is removed. The downside of the procedure is that, if too much disc is removed, the spinal segment can become unstable and a fusion surgery may be required soon after. There are many differing opinions regarding this procedure, but most mainstream spine surgeons do not perform it.

Lumbar Fusion

If you are told that lumbar fusion is the appropriate surgery for you, you may be suffering from lumbar degenerative disc disease, a recurrent disc herniation, lumbar spondylolisthesis, deformity, infection, or even cancer. Whatever the case may be, your spine surgeon is going to attempt to remove a disc and fuse bony segments to each other, which is similar to welding bones together in an attempt to stop any abnormal movement. A variety of different procedures is available and the way the spine is approached is different in each case. We must address several issues before discussing specific fusion procedures.

As previously discussed, the spine can be approached from the front or from the back. The front approach is called an anterior lumbar fusion, while an approach from the back is called a posterior lumbar fusion. An anterior approach allows surgeons to visualize the disc in its entirety and remove it completely. This will usually result in a higher fusion rate

if it is combined with a fusion posteriorly. Fusion performed posteriorly can be performed with or without metallic implants, but the use of
implants increases the success rate of fusion. Even though pedicle
screws were used some seventy years ago, they came into common use
only about fifteen years ago, as surgeons' skill in placing them safely
began to increase substantially. Pedicle screws are now the most common implant used to fuse sections of the spine.

As we mentioned in our earlier discussion of fusion surgery, synthetic protein known as bone morphogenetic protein (BMP), has been
introduced, increasing our success rate in achieving bony fusion. It is
relatively expensive, but widely available. This is good news for you if
you are planning to undergo such surgery. If your spine surgeon has
suggested proceeding with an anterior lumber fusion combined with a
posterior fusion, it may be referred to as a *360-degree fusion* or a *circumferential fusion* of your lower back. This is the most effective type of surgery available to achieve fusion of your lower back, but it is also the
most aggressive type of surgery performed. As previously suggested, it
requires two procedures, one performed through the anterior approach
and one through the posterior approach. Some spine surgeons will perform both of the procedures on the same day, while others prefer to perform the surgeries on different days. In most cases, your spine surgeon
will team up with a general or vascular surgeon, since vascular surgeons
routinely perform these types of procedures and are specialized in making the approach to, and exposing, the spine. Once the approach to the
spine is made, the spine surgeon removes the entire disc.

To fill the space from which the disc was removed, different materi-
als are available. Options include donated bone, special carbon material,
or a metallic implant. If your surgeon chooses donated bone, it is usually in the shape of a disc that can easily be placed in the empty disc space.
If a metallic implant is chosen, an array of shapes is available, each with
an associated theory as to why it is superior. No one implant, however,
has been shown conclusively to be better than the others.

The anterior approach allows your surgeon to increase the height of
the disc space. This will in turn increase the size of the neural foramen
(the exit zone of the nerves) at that level. By increasing the disc space, the
surgeon can indirectly decrease some pressure over the exiting nerves

and reduce your leg pain. The anterior approach also provides good visualization of the bone needed for fusion. Larger amounts of bone graft can be placed through the anterior approach as compared with the posterior. Either bone morphogenetic protein or bone removed from your pelvis can be placed in the area to increase the chance of a fusion.

Some spine surgeons perform this type of fusion without supplementation by posterior fusion. As I mentioned, however, we have seen higher failure rates for anterior fusion performed without posterior fusion, so most spine surgeons approach the spine posteriorly after performing a fusion anteriorly. If your spine surgeon has chosen to perform an anterior fusion along with a posterior fusion, you will be turned around to your abdomen to complete the surgery once the anterior surgery is done. During the posterior approach, the fusion can be supplemented and a decompression procedure can also be performed if necessary. Bone can easily be removed from the pelvis if needed as a bone graft. To increase the chances of fusion, pedicle screws or other metallic implants can be placed to keep the area immobile, which will allow your body to fuse the bone.

In recent years we have seen many spine surgeons begin to perform surgery using a variety of minimally invasive techniques. Your spine surgeon can avoid muscle stripping and damage by using percutaneous pedicle screws, which can be placed through multiple small incisions. If you are a candidate for a minimally invasive fusion approach, your expected recovery time is shorter and the risk of infection is lower. However, as with any type of spine surgery, risk of bleeding and damage to your nerves cannot be completely avoided. The minimally invasive fusion technique is also more technically demanding and poses more difficulty in the placement of bone graft. The risk of pseudarthrosis may be higher, as well.

Many different techniques exist to accomplish a lumbar fusion. Therefore, I will next describe each technique separately.

Anterior Lumbar Interbody Fusion (ALIF). This is a complicated surgery. We'll touch on the highlights here. The surgery is commonly performed along with a vascular surgeon who is specifically trained in exposing the spine for the spine surgeon. There are many important structures that reside in front of the spine. The surgeons first encounter the abdominal muscles, then the intestines, which are pushed to the side. Then they come across some extremely large blood vessels, which the vascular surgeon moves in order to expose the spine. In the event that one of these blood vessels is torn during surgery, the vascular surgeon has the specialized training to repair the damaged blood vessel. Such damage is the main risk of this surgery. In rare events, inability to repair the blood vessel can result in massive blood loss, which is a very dangerous situation. For this reason, most spine surgeons will use a machine called a Cell Saver to avoid massive blood loss during surgery. The Cell Saver suctions the blood, processes it, and returns it to the body.

Once the spine is exposed, special retractors are placed to keep the blood vessels and other important structures out of the way until the surgery is completed. The offending disc is confirmed, using an X-ray, and is then completely removed with specialized instruments. Spine surgeons call this *radical discectomy*. You end up with an empty space where the disc used to be. If you are having a fusion, some bone can be removed from the vertebra to create a smooth surface to the bone. In contrast, if you are having an artificial disc inserted in place of your own disc, it is extremely important to avoid removal of any bone so that the implant can sit correctly. Whatever implant your spine surgeon has chosen, it can then be placed relatively easily.

In each case, extreme care must be given to placement of the implant. It must be placed in the center of the disc space and bone graft or BMP should be supplemented to increase the chances of fusion. Different implants have various requirements and the manufacturer will offer specific placement techniques. In some cases, metallic implants can be placed in front of the disc implant to avoid movement of the implant to increase chances for fusion. Attention should be paid by your spine surgeon to avoid irritation of the major vessels near these metallic implants.

Posterior Lumbar Fusion (PLF). Posterior lumbar fusion can be performed by itself, or combined with a laminectomy, a laminotomy, or an anterior fusion. Furthermore, many different techniques are available for performing this surgery. Twenty years ago there was some controversy surrounding the use of metallic implants with this type of surgery, but today, most spine surgeons use some type of metallic implant when attempting to fuse the spine posteriorly.

The surgery is performed with you lying on your abdomen. In posterior lumbar fusion surgery, there is no need to team up with a vascular surgeon. Most of the bleeding comes from the muscles and, if bleeding occurs, it can easily be stopped. The muscles are moved to the side and the bone is exposed. Most surgeons will harvest bone from the pelvis to use as a bone graft later in the procedure. If you and your surgeon have also decided to perform a laminectomy or a decompression along with the fusion, it is performed prior to the completion of the fusion. The lamina is then removed and the nerves are freed from any pressure surrounding them. If SSEP monitoring is used, an improvement in the values can be seen following the decompression.

Next, the transverse processes (structures to the sides of the bones) are exposed to prepare the area for bone graft placement. This is the area that will house the fusion bone, once the fusion is completed. Upon exposure of the transverse processes, the hard outer shell of the bone, referred to as the *cortical bone,* is removed in a process called *decortication,* exposing the inner, spongy bone called *cancellous bone.* The cancellous bone fuses better and exposing it will increase the likelihood of bony fusion at the surgical site. Your surgeon will then place pedicle screws, which pass through the pedicles and into the vertebral body anteriorly. The placement of the screws requires experience and knowledge of detailed anatomy by your spine surgeon. Only a few millimeters separate each screw from nerves, so misalignment of the screw can damage a nerve in the surrounding area.

Once the screws are placed, they are attached to each other with connecting rods, which results in a very strong construct that will hold the bones to each other and stop any movement in the area. This rigidity will be the foreground to the formation of a bony fusion mass. The bone graft is then placed over the transverse processes. The screws will continue to keep the vertebrae from moving until the new bone is formed between them. This process will take anywhere from three to six months. Once the new bone is formed and a solid fusion mass is seen, the metallic implants will no longer be needed. This type of fusion does not address a fusion to the spine anteriorly but there are variations to this technique that allow a fusion in the disc space anteriorly, through the same incision.

Posterior Lumbar Interbody Fusion (PLIF) and Transforaminal Lumbar Interbody Fusion (TLIF). PLIF and TLIF are variations on the posterior fusion surgery. These procedures were developed to fuse the anterior section of the spine as well as the posterior section to achieve a 360-degree fusion, or the so-called circumferential fusion. As I mentioned in the section on anterior lumbar fusion, the traditional circumferential fusion is performed in two sessions. The surgery is first performed through the abdomen as an ALIF (see page 77) and supplemented with a posterior fusion. With the PLIF and TLIF, there is no need for your surgeon to approach the spine anteriorly. In order to fuse the spine circumferentially, the disc must be removed and the vertebral bodies fused. TLIF and PLIF accomplish the removal of the disc and fusion of the vertebrae through the posterior approach. This eliminates the risks to the vascular and internal structures of the abdomen that exist in the ALIF. This benefit is exchanged, however, for higher risks to the neural structures.

The approach to both of these procedures is the same. Through the posterior, the incision is made in the midline and the bony surface of the spine is exposed. The PLIF surgery uses a laminectomy with removal of bone and some of the facet joint. The dura and the nerve within the spinal canal are moved to the center. The disc is then visualized and a half-inch hole is made within the surface of the disc (the annulus). Using special instruments, the surgeon removes as much of the disc tissue as possible. It is not as easy to remove the disc through the posterior approach as it is through the anterior approach. The removal of the disc is performed through a very small opening in the disc space. At all times, the dura and the nerve adjacent to the dura are retracted to the side. This is one of the dangers of this surgery. Too much retraction can damage the nerve or the dura.

After the disc is removed, a small metallic implant or donated bone is placed in the disc space to stimulate the fusion of the vertebral bones. With PLIF, an implant is placed on each side of the spine, which requires extra dissection. Local bone graft from the laminectomy bone or bone harvested from the pelvis is placed within the disc space along with the implant. This will stimulate more aggressive bone formation to fuse the spine. At that time, pedicle screws are placed and the surgery is finalized in a fashion similar to the posterior fusion I described earlier.

Transforaminal lumbar interbody fusion (TLIF) is a variation of PLIF. In TLIF surgery, the entire facet joint is removed from one side. As we've discussed, the facet joint is the small joint connecting the vertebrae to each other in the back of the spinal column. Since the segment is being fused, the facet joint is no longer needed, and its removal allows good access to the disc space. The facet joint is the roof of the neural foramen. By removing the facet joint, your surgeon is placed directly within the neural foramen, which gives us the name of this procedure. After removal of the entire facet joint, wide access to the disc is possible and the posterior surface (the annulus) can easily be seen. The access to the disc space is wider and the disc can be removed more efficiently than in the PLIF procedure. Furthermore, your surgeon does not have to move the dura and the adjacent nerve as much as in the PLIF procedure. With TLIF, the risk to the neural structures is therefore lower than in the PLIF procedure. A larger implant can be placed in the disc space, since the opening to the disc space is larger than in the PLIF. In the TLIF, the dissection into the disc space is only from one side, further reducing the surgical risk and the length of the procedure. Since the opening into the disc space is larger, your surgeon has a better chance to elevate a collapsed disc space. Elevation of the disc space increases the size of the neural foramen, which indirectly releases pressure on any compressed nerves. The best chance to elevate the disc space, however, is with the ALIF procedure.

Even though there are advantages and disadvantages to each procedure, my opinion is that the TLIF procedure is superior to the PLIF procedure. PLF alone (see page 78) has the lowest chance of resulting in a solid fusion of the vertebrae, but it also exposes you to the lowest risk. Table 4.1 compares the risks and benefits of the four types of lumbar fusion we have discussed.

The technical ability of your surgeon, however, is, of course, one of the most important factors to consider in choosing which procedure is the right one for you. Even if one type of surgery is more beneficial for your problem, your spine surgeon may not be well trained in performing a specific type of technique. If your surgeon is not trained in the specific type of surgery, attempting to perform it may be more harmful than beneficial.

TABLE. 4.1. COMPARISON OF THE ASSOCIATED RISKS AND ADVANTAGES OF FOUR LUMBAR FUSION TECHNIQUES				
PROPERTIES	**ALIF**	**PLF**	**TLIF**	**PLIF**
Risk to vascular structures	xxxx	x	xx	xx
Risk to neural structures	xx	xx	xx	xxxx
Ability to elevate the disc space and decompress nerves indirectly	xxxx	—	xx	x
Requires approach through the abdomen	xxxx	—	—	—
Requires approach through the back muscles	—	xxxx	xxxx	xxxx
Ability to fuse the spine	xxxx*§	xx	xxx	xxx

* When combined with a posterior fusion
§ Fusion rates comparable to posterior fusion if performed as stand-alone anterior fusion.

Minimally Invasive Fusions. Even though the variety of procedures may be confusing, I have to introduce another twist to the story! All of the above procedures can be performed in a minimally invasive way and I will discuss some of the highlights next.

Anterior lumbar interbody fusion, as we have seen, uses an approach through the abdomen. The minimally invasive approach was to use a *laparoscopic* technique and perform the surgery through several small incisions in the abdomen. A few years back, however, some patients encountered catastrophic complications with massive bleeding. Due to these reported complications, minimally invasive anterior lumbar interbody fusion has been abandoned by most spine surgeons.

There have been many advances in recent years with minimally invasive TLIF and PLIF procedures. We are able to place pedicle screws percutaneously without the need to make long incisions and decompress the nerves, as I described in the section on minimally invasive microdiscectomy procedures. Using the same tubular retractors, the TLIF and PLIF procedures can be performed through a one-inch incision and pedicle screws placed percutaneously. This requires advanced training on the part of your spine surgeon and, unfortunately, not all spine surgeons have been trained in such techniques. Remember that not all procedures performed with minimally invasive techniques are necessarily the best choices. It depends on the specific condition you have, and the clinical scenario. If you require fusion in multiple spinal segments, performing the procedure with a minimally invasive technique may not be feasible and the ultimate decision will be up to your spine surgeon.

Lumbar Artificial Disc Replacement (ADR) Surgery. The theoretical benefit of ADR over lumbar fusion surgery is that the abnormal disc is removed without the need to fuse a disc level, allowing preservation of motion in that spinal segment. If you have a lumbar fusion, you incur a small risk that the disc next to the fused level can degenerate more rapidly. Some studies indicate that the risk is as low as 1 percent, while other studies indicate that it is as high as 20 percent. It is also known that degeneration can occur with or without fusion surgery next to a degenerated disc. ADR was introduced in an attempt to avoid this possible complication of lumbar fusion surgery.

ADR has been performed in Europe for many years, but the technology was not introduced in the United States because of the reservations of the Food and Drug Administration, which must approve the implant for general use in the United States. The first ADR approved for use in the United States was the Charité artificial disc from DePuy Spine Inc. (www.charitedisc.com), which calls the Charité the world's first artificial disc. The Charité disc was approved for transplantation in the lumbar spine, over one level only. The ideal candidate to receive this implant should not have instability or arthritis in the facet joint. The placement of the implant over two disc levels is not approved by the FDA but can be performed at the discretion of your surgeon. Most spine surgeons would not place the implant over three disc levels.

For a surgeon to have permission to implant this device in a patient, she is required to complete a course in order to understand the technique and theory behind it. Upon introduction of the implant, most spine surgeons were very enthusiastic about the potential benefits and many surgeons completed the course. Unfortunately, mixed opinions surfaced about the implant, for reasons of design, theory, and function. Some patients reported an excellent outcome, while others reported worsening of pain and dysfunction, and many catastrophic complications occurred. Soon, growing skepticism developed on the part of many surgeons and insurance companies because of these complications. For this reason, the number of ADR surgeries did not climb to expected levels.

One of the reasons for the lack of success of ADR is the fact that adjacent disc degeneration was never conclusively proven. The precise mechanism is not understood, since adjacent level degeneration may actually occur even in patients who have not had fusion of a spinal segment. Because of that, the theory explaining the advantage of ADR over lumbar fusion surgery is not clear.

The placement of an artificial disc uses the same surgical approach as an anterior lumbar fusion. The approach and the surgical dissection have been fully described. Most spinal surgeons are familiar with this approach, since anterior lumbar fusion is a common procedure. If the artificial disc is not placed appropriately, however, it can dislodge from the disc space and move into the abdomen. If the dislodged implant places pressure over the large vascular structures of the abdomen, it can cause pain, dysfunction of other body functions, and even death. Two to three weeks after an anterior abdominal surgery is performed, a great deal of scar tissue forms at the surgical site and around all the blood vessels within the surgical field. If an artificial disc is dislodged, returning to the operative site in the anterior spine could be a very difficult and risky operation. Rarely would a spine surgeon return to remove the artificial disc if it dislodges, breaks, or loosens. The accepted method of salvage for this operation is to attempt to fuse the spine from a posterior approach. Unfortunately, once an artificial disc is placed anteriorly, this task becomes much harder. If the disc is dislodged and places pressure over vital organs, the spine surgeon will be forced to attempt to return to the anterior spine, and remove the malfunctioning disc. This can be a risky undertaking, since scar tissue is very hard to maneuver and can result in brisk and risky bleeding that can be difficult to control.

Another disc—the Prodisc—was recently introduced by Synthes and approved by the FDA for use in the United States. The theory behind both of the implants is similar, though Synthes claims that the Prodisc is better designed and that the failures that were seen with Charité will be avoided by the Prodisc implant. Unfortunately, new complications are surfacing with this implant, even though the design may in fact be an improvement over the Charité implant.

If you are suffering from back pain and your surgeon has offered you a fusion surgery, disc replacement may be another option. The indications for ADR are much narrower, however, than for lumbar fusion surgery. Today, most spine surgeons will still recommend lumbar fusion surgery over ADR. This is because the loss of motion from a fusion surgery may not be significant. Your ability to bend forward and pick up objects from the floor comes from the hip joint and not the lumbar spine. ADR may not result in a better range of motion as compared to lumbar fusion surgery over one level. Salvage surgery is risky and can result in catastrophic complications.

Fortunately, the science behind spine surgery is rapidly evolving. You should get updated information about new techniques and implants from your spine surgeon, along with all of the options that may be available to you. For this reason, you should make sure that your spine surgeon is knowledgeable about the most advanced implants and techniques to treat your back condition.

Vertebroplasty and Kyphoplasty

If you are one of the many people who have suffered from an insufficiency or compression fracture of your spinal bones, you may be a candidate for kyphoplasty or vertebroplasty. Fractures that result from low bone density, or *osteoporosis*, are very common. They result in the collapse of the vertebral body, and in some cases cause severe pain. The idea behind these procedures is to inject cement into the bone. As the cement hardens, it produces heat in the area, which can theoretically burn the very small nerves in the bone that transmit the sensation of pain to your brain. The hardened cement also provides stability to the fractured bone and reduces pain dramatically. The procedure is performed by making a needle-hole size incision and placing a *trocar*—a shaft that is sharply pointed and usually three-sided—into the bone.

Vertebroplasty is a procedure in which cement is injected into the collapsed bone. There is no attempt to elevate the bone. The risk of vertebroplasty is that the cement can spread over the nerves and can place a lot of pressure on the nerves. This has the potential to cause catastrophic complications. For this reason, not many doctors perform this procedure anymore. *Kyphoplasty* has a lower risk of complications and can also elevate and restore the shape of the collapsed bone. The procedure is performed through a similar type of an incision with a trocar. With the placement of the trocar, a small balloon is passed inside the bone. The balloon is inflated, which restores the height of the collapsed bone. As the height of the vertebral body is increased, a space is produced in the shape of the balloon. The balloon is then removed and cement is injected within that space. Since an empty space is made, less pressure is needed to place the cement within the bone, which also decreases the risk of the cement seeping out and spreading over the nerves. As the cement hardens, heat is produced and destroys the small nerves that transmit pain sensation to the brain. Since the incision size is very small, the chance of infection is also very low. Kyphoplasty is the preferred procedure for compression fractures of the spine.

Even though the procedure is usually successful, you should try nonoperative treatment for about six weeks before proceeding with the surgery. Most compression fractures heal within a few weeks and the pain resolves with the use of a brace. There is something else to think about regarding this procedure: the fact that it increases the risk of fractures in the adjacent vertebral levels. In most cases, however, this procedure is successful and relatively easy. You should expect a one-day hospital stay and a relatively fast recovery from the surgery.

*   *   *

After all the time that went into learning about your back and your back problem, and then weighing the risks of surgery, it may have seemed rather simple to learn about each individual procedure. That's just what I was hoping! Next, we'll take a look at how you can best prepare for either inpatient or outpatient surgery, including choosing your surgeon and care facility.

PART TWO

Before and After Your Back Surgery

INTRODUCTION

Whether you are already committed to undergoing back surgery or are still undecided, it makes perfect sense that you are experiencing anxiety. What must you do prior to the procedure? How difficult will the recovery be? What are the pain-relief options? Will you be in the hospital for a long time?

Chapter 5 fills you in on the preparations for surgery. You have lots to consider, from what to look for in a surgeon to what type of facility you will need. And then there's the pre-surgery protocols, such as taking medications for other existing health concerns; being psychologically stable; and perhaps even storing blood in advance. It's time to think about these details, and this book will help you do so in a methodical, manageable way.

Then, breathe a sigh of relief. Let's imagine the surgery is done and you are coasting into recovery. Chapter 6 gives you the low-down on what to expect in the hours, days, and weeks after your procedure. Your expectations should be based on the type of anesthesia you were given and the pain management agenda you decide upon. There are also possible complications to discuss so that you never feel "in the dark" about what could happen. You will be guided through all of this so that you can approach your surgery with plenty of confidence and knowledge.

5

Preparing
for Surgery

Anxiety often accompanies back pain. You may feel uneasy that you can't perform certain tasks, or scared that you will miss work or important family affairs. If you thought that apprehension would disappear once you set your surgery date, you have probably learned that's not the case. If you are like most, you will have a reasonable amount of worry. Rest assured, this is normal. I'm so glad to be able to ease your concerns! In this chapter, we'll go step by step down the path of preparing for surgery. First, we'll talk about choosing your surgeon and hospital, and obtaining preoperative medical clearance. Then, we'll take a microscope to the ins and outs of inpatient and outpatient surgery.

CHOICES REGARDING YOUR
SURGEON AND CARE FACILITY

There is, of course, no definite or proven technique to insure that your surgery will be successful, or that your hospital stay will be pleasant. You can certainly increase your chances of success, however, if you are armed with knowledge. Undoubtedly, more effort should be put into choosing your physician than in choosing the hospital or other care facility. If you end up in a facility that is less than optimal, you may have a bad experience with the nurses, the service, the food, the bed, the room, or the atmosphere. This bad experience will last only for a limited time—a few days at most. On the other hand, if you choose a surgeon who is less than optimal, you could have bad results that will affect you for the rest of your life.

You may also find that, once you have chosen your surgeon, you will be limited to choosing from among the hospitals in which he has privileges. Most spine surgeons spend two-thirds of their time in the office and one-third in the hospital. They go to the hospital to perform surgery and to see their patients after surgery, and then return to the office to see patients. To decrease their commute time and have rapid access to their postoperative patients, their offices are usually located close to the hospitals with which they are affiliated.

Your Surgeon

There are two ways to find a spine surgeon. One is by the recommendation of your general doctor and the other is through your own investigation. Since the field of spine surgery is relatively specialized, you have probably been referred to a spine surgeon by your general physician, who most likely has a spine surgeon (or several) to whom he routinely refers. This referral pattern may be related to the proximity of his office to the spine surgeon's office or to his knowledge of the surgeon's work. Don't think, however, that this doesn't leave you any choice. In virtually every large city, there are many spine surgeons and you will have the option of choosing one from many. If you live in a smaller city or suburb, or if you reside in a rural area, you may have to travel to get to a surgeon. In almost every case, however, you will have a choice of surgeons.

The most important factor in deciding whether your spine surgeon is right for you is that you have a good relationship with him, including free-flowing communication. You should be able to communicate with your surgeon effectively and feel comfortable about your decisions. If there is any doubt in your mind regarding the type of surgery your spine surgeon has proposed or about issues such as the approach or the implant to be used, then you should consider obtaining a second opinion.

Training

The training of most spine surgeons includes four years of undergraduate studies, followed by another four years of medical school. From there, another five or six years of either orthopedic surgery or neurosurgery training is required. Depending on the region of the country, a one-year period is also required for training specifically in spine surgery. The most important element is the last year of training in spine surgery itself. This is usually called a fellowship. Your surgeon undergoes his most intense and concentrated period of learning during the spine surgery fellowship program. All of the education that preceded the fellowship program will be less significant. The undergraduate studies and the medical school education are almost irrelevant to the skills of your spine surgeon. Most of the education that your surgeon gets during an orthopedic or neurosurgery residency is in general principles of practice and basic surgical skills. Indeed, the training during residency is important, but not as crucial as the year of fellowship training. So, if you want to investigate your surgeon's education, look into the last year of his training.

Even though your search is now narrowed, it may get confusing! Some fellowship programs concentrate heavily on research and have limited clinical exposure. Other programs may concentrate intensively on clinical studies, including surgery of the spine. Obviously, your preference should be extensive clinical and surgical experience, as opposed to research activity. Unfortunately, there is no easy way to learn about the clinical exposure of your spine surgeon during his fellowship program. Even if you learn that a fellowship program has extensive clinical experience, it does not mean that your spine surgeon had extensive hands-on training. Some fellowship programs are associated with exclusive private practices that do not allow surgeons in training to practice their skills. These surgeons end up graduating without surgical skills and experience, although they may possess vast knowledge and have extensive visual exposure to many surgical procedures. You may want to ask your surgeon specifically about his training.

You should also ask him about the number of similar procedures he performs each month or year. It is important that your surgeon maintain a balance between being overly aggressive regarding surgery and being inexperienced. Too many surgical procedures may indicate that your surgeon is very aggressive in recommending surgery to his patients. Beware if your surgeon immediately recommends surgery. In almost all cases, spine surgery is elective and the choice to proceed with it is yours. There are only a few instances in which a surgeon should indicate that surgery is absolutely necessary. On the other hand, if your surgeon does not perform a particular procedure often enough, he may not be competent to perform your surgery. If he has performed a particular surgical procedure only once or twice before, be wary and reconsider your choice of surgeon!

Board Certification

Board certification is another important factor to examine when choosing a surgeon. As with most other subjects, here, too, there are exceptions and challenging issues. The basic concept is that there are two main legitimate boards—the American Board of Orthopaedic Surgery (www.abos.org) and the American Board of Neurological Surgery (www.abns.org). Both of these boards are part of a larger institution called the American Board of Medical Specialties (www.abms.org). Surgeons who are board certified enjoy a higher level of respect and trust from hospitals, insurance carriers, and other physicians.

The process of board certification starts after the completion of residency or a fellowship program. A written test is administered and, if it is completed successfully, the candidate becomes "board eligible." From there, the candidate must document information about every patient he treats surgically for a period of six months. A second test is administered about two years later and the candidate is orally questioned to examine the judgment, ethics, and clinical skills he has exercised in treating these patients. The oral test is administered by seasoned surgeons within that specialty. This strict and extensive testing helps insure that a physician is competent and possesses adequate knowledge. Once your surgeon is board certified, he will have the obligation to remain certified. The American Board of Orthopaedic Surgery requires recertification every ten years. This assures that your board-certified surgeon will stay up-to-date with the developing technology and science of spine surgery. If your surgeon is not board certified, there is no requirement to pursue further knowledge or training.

In addition to the American Board of Orthopaedic Surgery and the American Board of Neurological Surgery, there are lesser known, less legitimate boards that will certify almost any surgeon without the strict criteria to insure competence. Certification by unknown boards is relatively easy and is often sought by surgeons who were unable to get certification from the two legitimate boards.

Type of Practice

Another consideration in choosing your surgeon is the type of medical practice he has. Once your surgeon completes the required training, he will have to make a decision regarding the type of practice to start. Some surgeons will choose to begin their practice in an academic setting such as a large university hospital. Some decide to go into private practice, which can be either a group or solo practice. The decision to go into an academic setting or private practice depends solely upon the discretion of the surgeon and neither pattern of practice points to better technical skills or knowledge.

For a surgeon to enter an academic setting early in his career is relatively straightforward. Academic institutions provide all the necessities to start a practice. This includes the finances and the office structure, as well as the patients who need treatment. In return, the academic institution requires that the surgeon teach, treat patients, and, in most cases, perform some research activities. The primary focus of the physician is to serve the goals of the institution, which may leave the concerns of the patients behind.

You may think that a physician in an academic setting would be more up-to-date on the most advanced techniques; that is usually untrue, however, since physicians in an academic setting are subject to the control of the institution in many ways. For budgetary reasons, for instance, some academic centers will not allow surgeons to use the most technically advanced instruments. Furthermore, the surgeons in these centers may be heavily involved in research activities and not as involved in clinical practice.

If, on the other hand, your surgeon has decided to enter the private practice arena, he will be required to handle the finances and marketing, and to provide superb patient care. The competition is fierce and patient care must be excellent in order to encourage other physicians to refer their patients to the practice. Unfortunately, not all surgeons in private practice are competent or superb. This is what sets the busy practices apart from the failing ones. A physician who provides good care will flourish, and the ones who provide less than that will struggle. Surgeons who are in private practice will routinely perform more surgical cases and are usually less involved in research activities.

In either case—that of an academic setting or a private practice—you should concentrate on finding out as much as you can about the knowledge and skills of the surgeons whom you are considering. Clearly, you have a lot of research to do. However, feeling totally confident in your surgeon is priceless.

Litigation

You will also want to investigate whether your surgeon has been involved in litigation, and, if so, how many times. Undoubtedly, some malpractice litigation is unavoidable. Many surgeons have a few malpractice claims on their records. Sixty percent of all physicians (including generalists) are sued at least once during their careers; the numbers for surgeons are higher. Some surgeons refuse to undertake risky surgery, while others will attempt to help any patient. The surgeons who attempt riskier surgery may be exposed to a higher number of malpractice lawsuits. You should be concerned, however, if your surgeon has more than an average number of claims—i.e., more than five—especially if he legally lost many of these cases.

Again, the Internet is a good source of information. Websites such as www.mdnationwide.org can provide some information about the malpractice history of a physician, but they will charge you for that information. It is important to note that these websites only provide information regarding lawsuits that resulted in a payoff from the insurance company. Information may be difficult to obtain regarding cases in which no payment was made by the insurance carrier on behalf of the physician. If a lawsuit is filed, but the case is closed without any payoff and therefore in favor of the physician, then no record may be available.

Insurance and HMO Plans

The type of insurance coverage you have will also affect your choice of surgeon. Even if you have health coverage under an HMO, however, you probably still have a choice among several spine surgeons. Do not shortchange yourself with uncertainty or limited knowledge because your health coverage is with an HMO.

In most cases, the knowledge and training of the physicians within the HMO system will not differ from surgeons outside that system. Unfortunately, the treatment that you receive may differ or the choice of hospitals that can be used during your surgery may be very limited. Remember that HMO systems were originally developed to minimize health-care costs. Today, this is still the goal of the HMO systems. If your health insurance coverage is through an HMO, your hospital stay will most likely be shorter, since much emphasis is placed by the HMO administrators on decreasing costs, which includes length of hospital stay. That should not affect your surgeon's decisions, however, regarding the type of surgery he recommends or the technique he proposes to use to perform your surgery.

Websites

In this case—if you are looking for a spine surgeon—the Internet may not be the most reliable source of information. Websites can be designed relatively easily by anyone, and the quality of the website will largely depend on the amount of money spent to create it.

Remember that generally the contents of websites are not controlled by any specific agency or authority. Flashy websites may seem more impressive at first glance; many of them, however, are created by giant implant companies and are therefore not representative of all viewpoints. The websites that are built by the implant companies tend to be more generic and to avoid detailed information out of fear of legal actions. Impressive illustrations and elaborate descriptions will be available on expensive implants, with a dearth of information on simple procedures that do not require implants. The more reliable websites are instead often created by surgeons themselves.

Two particular websites, however, are worth visiting. The websites of the American Academy of Orthopaedic Surgeons (www.aaos.org) and the North American Spine Society (www.spine.org) are the most respected websites in this health field. There is unbiased information on these sites.

The Facility

After you have made a decision about your spine surgeon, the decision about the hospital may not be as difficult. Since I am unable to write about specific hospitals and facilities, I will discuss the different types of facilities, including outpatient or ambulatory surgery centers (ASCs), specialty hospitals, and academic hospitals. I am confident you are already familiar with community hospital and major hospital environments; they are traditional hospital settings. Most major spine surgery will be done in a hospital setting. The more minor procedures can be performed in either a hospital or a facility that does not have the capacity to keep patients overnight. These include the outpatient or ambulatory surgery centers.

Outpatient or Ambulatory Surgery Centers (ASCs)

Outpatient and ambulatory surgery centers (ASCs) have flourished in recent years. The terms are often used interchangeably. The number of ASCs has grown hand in hand with the development of minimally invasive procedures. As we have seen, these procedures have been popularized, since they promote smaller incisions—or even no incision—which results in faster recovery that does not require a hospital stay after surgery. Complicated, risky, or lengthy operations cannot be done in an ASC because ASCs cannot provide blood transfusions and are not equipped with a radiology center if complications arise requiring more diagnostic studies. Furthermore, ASCs are only equipped with instruments that are needed to perform specific types of surgery.

Even considering all these limitations, however, a large percentage of surgical procedures are performed at ASCs because of the many benefits that ASCs offer. ASCs are often very convenient for doctors. The facilities are architecturally well planned and many are built adjacent to doctors' offices. Many doctors feel that the management of the ASC has better control over their employees, which results in a more efficient working environment. In comparison to hospitals, ASCs are dedicated to a few special procedures, which results in efficiency and simplicity. This is very important to surgeons, who wish to save time in performing their procedures. Scheduling is also simpler and faster with ASCs. Major hospitals are usually crowded, and scheduling a surgical procedure can be difficult, since many surgeons schedule procedures weeks in advance. Surgeons often have to change their schedules to accommodate the time that was provided to them by the hospital operating room. This creates inconvenience for many surgeons and pushes them toward scheduling their procedures in an ASC.

Pain management procedures such as discograms, epidural injections, facet blocks, and IDET procedures are the most common spine procedures performed at ASCs. They can be performed rapidly, which makes them most suited for an ASC. Operations that can be performed in an ASC include microdiscectomies, minimally invasive discectomies, and anterior cervical discectomies and fusions. Very few ASCs are set up for the performance of anterior lumbar fusions or fusion surgery that requires the implantation of metallic implants. The last two procedures are lengthy operations that usually require a hospital stay after the surgery. Occasionally, they also require blood transfusions. Should complications occur, other specialized instruments that may or may not be available in the ASC might be required.

ASCs that perform the more elaborate procedures are usually affiliated with rehabilitation centers that can provide further monitoring after the surgery. Some ambulatory surgery centers and outpatient surgery centers can keep you for twenty-three hours after the surgery, but after the first twenty-three hours, they will have to send you home or to a rehabilitation center. The reason for this time constraint is that if they keep their patients for more than twenty-three hours, they will be acting as a hospital, which has different—much more stringent—legal requirements. In most cases, you will be able to talk to your surgeon about your preference for a particular type of facility. All spine surgeons have privileges at major hospitals and some will have privileges at an ASC. Don't be afraid to express your concerns about this subject.

Specialty Hospitals

Specialty hospitals can be seen as glorified ASCs or outpatient surgery centers. Specialty hospitals are facilities that provide specific types of services. A traditional hospital will have most routine services, such as obstetrics, radiology, surgery, internal medicine, emergency room, and some common specialty services. In contrast, a specialty hospital may provide only limited services for specific types of patients. Examples of these services are cancer surgery, orthopedic surgery, or spine surgery. Currently, the federal government is considering passing new laws regarding the viability of such specialty hospitals and the final decision regarding the survival of this type of institution is still pending. Specialty hospitals are generally well equipped and provide good surgical care in a safe environment to their patients. They do not provide emergency room services like other, more comprehensive, hospitals, and their resources are directed to nonemergency, elective patient care. Surgeons who practice in specialty hospitals are generally satisfied with the services of these facilities, which translates to patient satisfaction.

Academic Hospitals

Academic hospitals are generally very large institutions that provide medical care in multiple specialties. These hospitals are usually involved in research and in house residency and training programs. Benefits of these institutions include the availability of resident doctors around the clock and many doctors with specialty training. Usually, there is good cooperation between the specialty services, which can provide you with care if your illness is complicated and requires coordination between physicians of different specialties. An example of such a scenario might involve a patient who has cancer or an infection of the spine.

The downside of the academic centers is that the majority of routine care is provided by physicians who are still in training and are under the supervision of attending surgeons. Parts of your surgery may be performed by residents in training and not by the surgeon who you expected to perform your surgery. As compared with a surgeon in an academic setting, a surgeon in a private hospital usually performs the procedure that you need on a routine basis—that is, multiple times in a month. There are no data, however, suggesting that the operative results in an academic center are inferior to the results of a private practicing surgeon. After all, the goal of any physician is to get good results and favorable outcomes for his patients.

YOUR PREOPERATIVE MEDICAL CLEARANCE

Wherever your surgery is scheduled to be performed, your surgeon will require a medical clearance prior to your surgery. Unless your procedure is a minor one, your body will be stressed during the surgery. In order to decrease operative risk, your internal organs will have to be checked to see whether your body can handle the stress of surgery. Consider your medical clearance like a tune-up of your car before a long trip. If you have asthma, diabetes, congestive heart failure, or hypertension, your internist can optimize your medical condition to decrease the risk of complications during surgery.

Your surgeon will ask you to schedule your preoperative medical clearance with a general physician one or two weeks before your surgery. If you have medical conditions that increase your surgical risk, the appointment may be set earlier so that enough time is allowed for specialized testing and appropriate treatment. Routine medical clearance testing includes blood work, an electrocardiogram (EKG), and a chest X-ray. If you are a woman in your childbearing years and are sexually active, you should have a pregnancy test to insure that you are not pregnant. The medications used during the administration of anesthesia may be detrimental to a fetus in the womb.

If you have other medical conditions, you may require more extensive testing of your lungs, heart, or liver. Tests such as an echocardiogram, a cardiac stress test, and a pulmonary function test are among those you may require if your risk for the surgery is higher. Your internist will prepare a summary of your evaluation through a report addressed to your surgeon and anesthesiologist. Your anesthesiologist will rely on that report and will adjust your medications according to your medical history and your medical condition. In most cases, anesthesiologists and general physicians who provide the medical clearance are in agreement with each other. Occasionally, an anesthesiologist may disagree with the opinion of the generalist, and, in these instances, the opinion of the anesthesiologist supersedes that of the generalist. That is because the ultimate responsibility lies on the shoulders of the anesthesiologist once you are asleep and anesthetized during surgery.

PREPARATIONS FOR SURGERY

The preparation for your surgery depends on whether the surgery is outpatient or inpatient. Simpler procedures are usually performed on an outpatient basis, while more involved surgical procedures are performed on an inpatient basis. A few principles are common to both. You should not eat or drink anything after midnight the day before your surgery. The reason is that you may vomit under anesthesia if there is food in your stomach. Even fluids are forbidden, except a little water to take essential medications. Also, you should review any existing health conerns with your physician. Some concerns are discussed in the next section.

Existing Health Problems

Many back surgery patients are already on certain types of medications and have dietary requirements due to existing health problems. If you are in this position, it is crucial that you discuss well in advance with your physician any medications and/or supplements that you routinely take, as well as any concerns you may be experiencing. Diabetes, hypertension, and asthma are three very common conditions that necessitate special attention.

Diabetes

If you are diabetic, it will be more difficult for you not to eat or drink anything prior to surgery. Your blood sugar may fluctuate more, and some surgeons will choose to perform your surgery first thing in the morning if you are diabetic. Close monitoring and control of your blood sugar are essential, since surgery can radically increase your blood sugars. In most cases, your surgeon will instruct you to keep taking your diabetic medications, except on the day of surgery, when you are not eating any food. If you don't eat yet take your diabetes medication, your blood sugar may plummet dangerously. In that case, you might feel light-headed or anxious, or you might develop other medical complications that could necessitate the cancellation of your surgery.

Hypertension

You should never skip your antihypertension medications. Maintaining a normal blood pressure is important for several reasons. First, an elevated blood pressure can increase bleeding during surgery. It makes it much more difficult for your surgeon to work when there is excessive bleeding in the surgical wound. High blood pressure can also increase the risk of bleeding after your surgery. In the case of surgery to the spine, postoperative bleeding around the spinal cord can cause devastating complications. Second, surgery by itself can increase your blood pressure, and that can increase your risk for a stroke or a heart attack. Skipping even one dose of your blood pressure medication can abnormally raise your blood pressure. If you have unusually high blood pressure, your surgeon or your anesthesiologist may cancel your surgery until your blood pressure is better controlled. If you have questions regarding which medications you should and should not take, ask your physician. The recommendations provided here are only guidelines and specific information should be provided by your own doctor.

Asthma

If you suffer from asthma—a common condition—your breathing and lung function should be closely monitored. Pulmonary function tests are routinely performed before surgery, and, if needed, appropriate medications can decrease wheezing and congestion. Bronchitis and other lung conditions should be aggressively treated to avoid complications during and after the surgery.

Steroids

Use of steroids is another issue to consider before surgery. *Cortisone* is a type of chemical that your body naturally produces in response to stress, in order to regulate many different processes. Cortisone is also used as a medication for a variety of conditions such as lupus, asthma, bronchitis, and rheumatoid arthritis. This is also the medication used in epidural injections. Many orthopedic surgeons inject joints with cortisone if inflammation and pain are diagnosed. Cortisone reduces inflammation by slightly weakening your immune system. Unfortunately, it can delay the healing of your wounds after the surgery and may slightly increase your chances of getting a wound infection. Extra efforts should be made to prevent infection if you have taken steroids for extended periods before the surgery.

Steroid medications taken on a long-term basis also suppress the natural ability of your body to release steroids during times of stress, like surgery. For this reason, your internist may suggest taking an extra dose of steroids right before the procedure to prepare your body for the stress that is inevitable with any type of operation. Based upon the recommendation of your general physician, your anesthesiologist will administer the steroids immediately before the surgery.

Diet

After any surgery, your body will need to heal and recover. This recovery period demands energy and protein to build new cells required in the healing process. Lack of adequate nutrition has been shown to increase complications after surgery, including infection. Malnutrition is common in the elderly and must be actively avoided. Though there is no doubt that overeating and obesity are detrimental to your health, you should avoid excessive dieting before your surgery. Eat normally and, at least a few days before the procedure, indulge in the foods that you like, especially those that are higher in protein content. Increasing your protein intake before surgery will decrease your chances for complications such as infection or wound-healing problems. Energy and protein are plentiful in food.

You will have plenty of opportunity to diet after your surgery. For starters, you may not have access to foods that you like. Unfortunately, pain and medications can suppress your appetite. And finally, the food in most hospitals is not appetizing, since more emphasis is placed on the quantity of the food than on its taste. I usually encourage the families of my patients to bring food from home, which makes my patients happy and allows their families to take an active role in their recovery.

Hygiene and Other Concerns

If you have body hair in the area of the surgery, you should leave it alone and let the nursing staff take care of it in the operating room before the surgery. Even if you think you are relatively hairless, there is still very fine hair over your skin that will need shaving before surgery. If you think you can prepare better by shaving the area yourself, you are wrong. Studies have shown that shaving well in advance of surgery allows bacterial growth within the skin pores, which can increase the risk of infection. So, it is best to have a nurse shave the skin right before the surgery, after you have gone to sleep from the anesthesia.

If you don't take a shower before your surgery, you probably won't increase your risk for infection. Before surgery, the surgical site is meticulously cleaned by the nursing staff to decrease the risk of infection. There are new cleaning solutions that insure almost complete eradication of bacteria on your skin at the surgical site. Of course, it's just common courtesy to the surgical staff to be clean and well groomed before the surgery. So take a shower the night before or the morning of surgery. Avoid using any vitamin creams or lotions on the surgical area.

It's probably a good idea to get a haircut before the surgery. This is especially true if you are having major surgery that will require a hospital stay. If you are having an outpatient pain management procedure, a haircut before the surgery is not an issue you must think about; if you are having a lumbar fusion, however, you will probably need a few days in the hospital and you will not have a chance to wash your hair or your body. A short haircut can eliminate some of your hygiene concerns after the surgery.

It may seem like a minor issue, but perhaps you have wondered if you are going to be naked in front of the surgical staff. The answer is yes. But rest assured that the surgical staff is professional and you are not in the operating room to be judged by anyone. Everyone in the room is very busy preparing for the surgery and is not concerned about the way your body looks. In most cases, you will be covered by blankets or heating units, and the period that your body is exposed is very limited. The nurses and your surgeon are your advocates to take care of your needs during and after your surgery.

Psychological Preparation

Psychological preparation is another very important part of getting ready for your surgery. The best way to decrease your anxiety is by eradicating the unknowns. This means eliminating surprises and understanding the process you are about to undergo. This book is one resource for that purpose. There are many other resources available, such as the Internet, and, of course, your surgeon, who can inform you about the possible risks and outcomes, which will lessen your anxiety.

Avoid gathering information from your neighbors or friends who may have piecemeal knowledge of spine surgery. Many patients will ask a friend who went through surgery and will make their entire decision based on the experience of one person they know. This can be a mistake. The one person you are asking these questions may have had an uncommonly good or bad experience. You should also remember that your problems may be very different from those of the person with whom you are discussing your condition. Furthermore, as technology advances, the same surgical procedures performed a few years ago may no longer be performed, or may have been vastly improved; if you compare your surgery to someone else's, you should make sure you are comparing the same condition and type of surgery.

Undoubtedly, even when you think that you have gathered much information, you will still have some anxiety and fear. No good spine surgeon will give you any guarantees, but he can reassure you that he will do his best to get good results from your surgery. Risks always exist, however, and there is a small chance that your surgery will not go according to plan. This is what creates anxiety for most people. You should be able to attain some comfort from the fact that you have made the best possible decision based on the available information, and you have accepted the fact that some things will not be under your control.

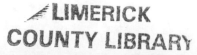

Remember that some anxiety is acceptable and even to be expected. Now may be a good time to take a class or listen to a tape instructing you in relaxation techniques like deep breathing, meditation, guided relaxation, visualization, or music therapy. You may be surprised by how much these simple self-help techniques can reduce your stress and anxiety—not only about your surgery, but about any other stressful areas of your life as well.

You may have trouble sleeping the night before the surgery, but, fortunately, it will not affect your surgical outcome. It is far more important that your surgeon get a good night's sleep, so set your worries aside and relax. Take comfort in the fact that many spine surgeries are performed daily, and in most cases the outcome is favorable. The risk of a catastrophic outcome is extremely low. Every imaginable complication can happen, as is the case with the simple act of walking across the street. At any moment, you can be hit by a car, but most people don't even think about the risk. Of course, no one can give you a guarantee that you will safely cross the street, but it's almost expected that nothing will happen, since the risk is relatively low. The same concept applies to spine surgery.

To avoid further anxiety, on the day of your surgery, remove your jewelry and valuables to avoid security issues during the surgery. The staff will have to make special arrangements for your valuables if you take them with you to the hospital. It is best to leave these with a family member or friend. If you were provided with a spinal brace to use after the surgery, take it with you and leave it with your companion. If you come alone, you can give your valuables or your brace to the surgical nurse, who will be looking after you throughout your surgery.

Advance Directives

Even though the risks of surgery are relatively low—and the risk of death or catastrophic complication is even lower—they still do exist. As a competent adult, you have the right to approve or deny any medical treatment. What happens, though, if you are no longer competent to make these decisions? As with any possible complications, you should always be prepared for the worst. Health-care advance directives are an essential tool you should consider signing before any surgical procedure. A living will and durable power of attorney for health care are two types of advance directives you can draw up before your surgery. These documents clearly provide information about your wishes for health-care treatment in case you are not able to make decisions on your own. You can also choose a health-care agent or proxy to make decisions on your behalf about your health. This person can be anyone close to you whom you trust to make appropriate decisions for you. Most people will choose their spouse, siblings, parents, or children. Resuscitation and the use of life-support machines to extend life are issues often handled by health-care agents. Other concerns may include the performance of further surgery to extend your life, while considering the quality of remaining life. These are sensitive and personal subjects that you should think about even if you are not having surgery.

Most hospitals offer information regarding these issues and have forms that you can fill out before your admission. The Internet is another resource that can be of help. The sites www.lawdepot.com, www.legacywriter.com, and www.abanet.org/aging/toolkit are only a few that you can use to draw up these documents. If you require a more personal service, many attorneys and social workers are available to draft these documents for you. An attorney will surely cost much more than the alternatives, however.

These documents can be stored in the hospital in case any questions arise at a later time. By storing the documents at a hospital, you can rest assured that the documents will be available in your chart should you ever need them again. They can be simply requested and even transferred to another hospital.

OUTPATIENT PROCEDURES

Outpatient procedures are relatively simple, and you are allowed to return home the same day as your surgery. These are usually simpler cases that do not require extensive dissection and result in mild to moderate postoperative pain. Almost all pain management procedures are also performed on an outpatient basis.

On the morning of your procedure, wear comfortable and loose clothing that you can take off easily. Afterward, you will need to put them back on; loose clothing is easy to put on and less likely to place pressure over the area of the procedure. The surgical facility will give you a gown that you will change into and most will have lockers in which to place your belongings before the surgery. Arrange for transportation and for help after the procedure. A close family member or friend can probably help you emotionally and can assist if any surprises arise during or after the surgery. Depending on the complexity of your procedure, your doctor may or may not request a medical clearance before you leave.

INPATIENT PROCEDURES

Procedures that require a hospital stay are called inpatient procedures. If your surgeon informed you that you will be staying in the hospital after your surgery, then your procedure is probably more involved, and you may require more potent pain medications after your operation. The requirement for close medical monitoring, a higher risk of needing a blood transfusion, or the necessity of rehabilitation are some of the other reasons you may stay in the hospital. As with any surgery, avoid taking anti-inflammatory medications a few weeks before the procedure. Anti-inflammatory medications can interfere with your platelet function and, as we have discussed, can result in increased bleeding during your surgery. It will be difficult for your surgeon to perform the operation if there is excessive bleeding in the surgical field. If you are having a spinal fusion surgery, it will be even more important to avoid anti-inflammatory medications. There is evidence that anti-inflammatory medications can decrease your chances of successfully fusing the necessary bones. It is generally accepted that you should stop taking anti-inflammatory medications a few months prior to spinal fusion surgery.

BLOOD TRANSFUSIONS

Some complex, lengthy procedures pose a higher risk for the necessity of a blood transfusion. The procedure that has the highest likelihood of requiring a blood transfusion is a lumbar fusion. If your surgery is complex or has an increased likelihood of requiring a blood transfusion, your surgeon may require that you donate your own blood prior to the procedure.

Blood consists of many different types of cells, and each type of cell has a specific task. The two main cell types are the white and red blood cells. The purpose of the white blood cell is to fight infections. The most abundant cells in the blood are the red blood cells, which have the task of carrying oxygen to the different organs in your body. The red blood cells can be regarded as delivery trucks and the oxygen can be regarded as food. There are a fixed number of trucks and a fixed number of locations to which the trucks must travel. If there are suddenly fewer trucks available to do the same work, the remaining trucks will have to travel faster to get to the same number of destinations. If there is blood loss, your organs will not receive enough oxygen, and your heart will begin to beat faster to circulate the limited available red blood cells throughout your body. You may feel fatigued and even anxious. Your doctor will be looking at your heart rate as one indication of the level of blood in your body.

Blood is needed for the proper functioning of your brain, kidneys, skin, bones, and every other organ. If your blood level is low, you will have a higher risk of developing an infection or having wound-healing problems. Critically low levels of blood can result in heart attacks, strokes, or even kidney failure. Having low levels of blood is similar to suffocating your organs. A simple blood test can tell your doctor about the level of blood in your body. A *complete blood count* (CBC) is the name of the test that is routinely used to check your blood level. A CBC will give an accurate count of your hemoglobin and hematocrit. Depending upon your age and medical history, your doctor can judge your need for a blood transfusion. If you are older, or have a history of heart disease, your doctor will have a lower threshold at which to give you a blood transfusion. A bad heart will not be able to cope with the need to beat very fast in case of low blood levels. For that reason, you may need a blood transfusion relatively quickly, as compared with a person who is young or a person who does not have heart disease. If you need aggressive rehabilitation, you may feel fatigued and your doctor may suggest a transfusion early on to prevent fatigue and expedite your recovery.

Autologous Blood Transfusion

There are multiple techniques that your surgeon can use to decrease the risks associated with a blood transfusion. The most common technique is *autologous blood transfusion*, or preoperative blood donation. With this technique, your surgeon will send you to the blood bank to donate your own blood before the surgery. In most cases, one unit of blood is donated every few weeks. The unit of blood is removed from your body and is sent for multiple tests. If it is evaluated to be safe, it is stored in the hospital until the time of surgery. Your body will detect the lower level of blood in your system, which is similar to blood loss, stimulating your body to produce new blood. Two or three units of blood can be donated, with the last unit being drawn about two weeks before the surgery. Your body will have enough time to naturally replenish the blood before the operation. If you require a blood transfusion during or after surgery, the blood that you donated before the surgery can be given right back to you.

This is found to be the safest type of transfusion, since it eliminates the risk of transmitting any diseases. Of course, the risk of human error, such as a labeling mistake, is not eliminated even with this type of transfusion. In recent years, much attention has been paid to human mistakes, and safeguards are in place to decrease human errors in many routine activities in hospitals around the nation.

Volunteer-Donated Blood

The other option, if you need a blood transfusion, is to obtain volunteer-donated blood from a blood bank. As you probably already know, one source of volunteer-donated blood is the American Red Cross. The American Red Cross arranges blood drives and collects blood from volunteers in the community. This form of blood transfusion has a higher risk of disease transmission than autologous blood donation, but the risk still remains extremely low. There is a rigorous screening program to decrease the chances of disease transmission. Each donor must answer multiple questions before being allowed to donate blood. The blood is then tested for multiple diseases, including HIV and hepatitis.

Even though rigorous testing is done on each unit of donated blood, the risk of disease transmission is not completely eliminated. As the tests become more sophisticated, the risk of disease transmission also decreases. The risk of getting an HIV infection from a blood transfusion is 1 in 700,000. The risk of getting a hepatitis infection is 1 in 3,000. You may want to compare that with the risk that you take every day when you cross the street or drive your car around town.

Directed Blood Donation

If these two options—using your own blood or volunteer-donated blood—are not appealing to you, other choices are available to reduce the risk of blood transfusions. You can choose the person you would like to donate blood to you. This is called *directed blood donation*. Of course, the blood type must match before you can choose to use that person's blood. Most people choose a close relative or their spouse as a directed donor. Even though you may think that blood from a directed donor is safer, it has not been shown to be safer than blood from a volunteer donor. This may be due to the fact that the same rigorous predonation screening is not performed with directed blood donation.

The Cell Saver

There are techniques that your surgeon can use to eliminate the need for a blood transfusion altogether. During surgery you may slowly bleed from the surgical wound and your surgeon will use a suction tube to remove that blood. Otherwise, your surgeon will not be able to see the important structures in order to perform the surgery. This blood can be delivered by the suction tube to a machine called a Cell Saver. This machine processes the blood that is lost during surgery so it can immediately be returned to your body in the operating room. Most major hospitals have a Cell Saver machine, and it is usually used in surgical cases where bleeding is expected. The Cell Saver cannot be used if you have cancer or infection. This is because the collected blood will have the bacteria or the cancer cells in it and returning the blood to your body can rapidly spread these cells throughout your body.

Hemodilution

Another interesting technique—one that is not routinely practiced—is called *hemodilution*. The idea behind this technique is to dilute your own blood by removing blood right before surgery and replacing it with fluids. If you lose some blood during surgery, you would lose blood that is diluted with fluids. The blood that was removed before the surgery can be transfused back into your body after the surgery, when the surgical bleeding has stopped. This technique can only be used if you are young and healthy, with good heart function. It can stress your heart, since the blood that is circulating is diluted and cannot carry oxygen as efficiently. For that reason, your heart has to pump the blood faster to deliver the oxygen to the different organs.

*   *   *

Now we've fully examined what it takes to get ready for surgery. In the next chapter we will look at what you can do to ease your pain and discomfort while expediting your recovery. Being prepared for the "after" effects will enhance your confidence and assuage anxiety.

6

Your Successful Recovery

Although you could not avoid the back problem that brought you to surgery, you can avoid pitfalls on the road to a successful recovery. Depending on what type of procedure and anesthesia you undergo, your immediate postoperative condition can vary substantially. I will begin by describing the different types of anesthesia that may be used so that you can understand the recovery from them more clearly.

TYPES OF ANESTHESIA

The two main categories of anesthesia are general anesthesia and regional anesthesia with sedation. Furthermore, there are three types of regional anesthesia: spinal anesthesia, epidural anesthesia, and local skin anesthesia.

General Anesthesia

The most common type of anesthesia is general anesthesia, which puts you into a deep, unconscious state. Special anesthetics and pain medications are injected into the intravenous catheter that is placed in your arm before the surgery. After about thirty seconds, you enter an unconscious state so deep that all your muscles will relax. A special machine known as a *ventilator* will breathe for you during the operation. It mixes oxygen with anesthetic gases, which are then delivered into your lungs through the breathing tube. The amount of medication is precisely controlled by your anesthesiologist, who will also monitor your vital signs.

After the operation is finished, your care will once again be turned over to your anesthesiologist. While your surgeon is removing her gown and gloves, your anesthesiologist will slowly wake you up from the anesthesia. Medications will be administered through your IV line to reverse the muscle paralysis that was induced at the beginning of your surgery. At the same time, your body will slowly get rid of the remaining anesthetic gases by having you exhale them from your lungs. After a short period of time, you will be able to breathe on your own and will become more conscious. In most cases, you will wake up in the operating room, although you may not recall this stage because of the residual effect of the anesthetics. The breathing tube that had been placed in your mouth will be removed once you have partially woken up. Most patients do not recall this part of the process, either.

Because general anesthesia is regarded as a relatively safe process, and it is widely available, most spine surgeons will choose to use general anesthesia for their patients. If you have certain types of heart or lung conditions that preclude you from having general anesthesia, however, your surgeon may consider the alternative local and spinal anesthesia to perform your surgery.

Regional Anesthesia

Regional anesthesia allows pain relief without placing your body in a state of complete paralysis and unconsciousness. With this type of anesthesia, you are awake but do not feel the area of the surgery. There are several advantages of regional anesthesia: a machine does not have to take over the breathing process for you; the body does not go into a state of unconsciousness, which results in greater stress on the heart; and the risk of pneumonia is lower. If you have a heart or lung condition, regional anesthesia is therefore a safer type of anesthesia.

Spinal Anesthesia

The use of spinal anesthesia is relatively limited in spine surgery. It is more commonly used in general orthopedic surgery, such as the repair of hip fractures or surgery on the legs. It is also routinely used when women deliver a baby through a caesarean section. With this technique, an anesthetic is injected into the fluid that bathes your spinal cord and the nerves in your lower spine. This anesthetizes and numbs the lower part of your spine, your abdomen, and your legs. The numbness slowly resolves after two hours. If you have this type of anesthesia, you are completely conscious and can hear and talk to your surgeon during the procedure. This type of anesthesia is considered safer in patients who have respiratory problems. The complications of spinal anesthesia are similar to those of epidural anesthesia; both are discussed in the next section.

Epidural Anesthesia

With epidural anesthesia, a tiny catheter is placed in the epidural space—the space between the bone and the nerves within your spinal canal—and the medications are administered through this tube. The advantage of this technique, like that of spinal anesthesia, is that you are not rendered unconscious and you keep breathing on your own. The potential complications of general anesthesia are avoided and there is less risk of a lung infection. The downside of these techniques is that you may move and may sometimes feel pain during surgery. Furthermore, this type of anesthesia is not desirable for procedures that require you to be either on your side or on your abdomen. It is very difficult to lie on your abdomen for too long, which can cause further discomfort, and increases the chance that you will begin to move around during surgery. Any movements you make during surgery can be dangerous and will render the work of your surgeon more difficult.

Skin Anesthesia

Superficial or skin anesthesia is usually used if you are getting an epidural injection, a facet injection, or a discogram. Since the skin is very sensitive to pain, your doctor will numb a small area of the skin with a thin needle (similar to the one used by a dentist). Because the needle used to numb the skin is so small, there is little pain when the anesthetic medication is injected into your skin. A few seconds after the injection, your skin will become so numb that you would not even be able to feel a stab with a scalpel. This type of anesthesia is used when wounds are sutured and when minor plastic surgery procedures are performed. Your doctor can then introduce a large needle through your skin without any pain or discomfort to you.

THE RECOVERY ROOM

The recovery room is the place that is equipped with the required personnel and instruments to help you wake up from the anesthesia. This area of the hospital can be intimidating, since there is usually a great deal of traffic and there are many gadgets and monitors. The task of the recovery room staff is to keep a close eye on you as you come out of the operating room and allow you to fully wake up from the anesthesia in a safe and controlled environment. In most cases, you will be kept in the recovery room for one or two hours, in order to insure stability of your vital signs and the absence of any unexpected bleeding from the wound. If your surgery was performed in a surgery center, the nurses should make sure that you are fully awake and medically stable before sending you home. In a hospital setting, you are likely to be moved into a regular room for the rest of your hospital stay, after getting clearance from the recovery room.

Each recovery bed will have a dedicated monitor that shows your heart rate, blood pressure, and the level of oxygen in your blood. The heart rate is measured by placing electrical stickers on your chest. These are attached to wires that are connected to a monitor, which will then interpret how fast your heart is beating and whether there are any abnormalities in your heartbeat. The heart rate is very important, since abnormalities in it may be one of the first signs of a complication. Excessive and abnormal bleeding or an unusually high level of pain can lead to increased heart rate and a drop in blood pressure. Elevated blood pressure can also point to excessive pain. An abnormally slow heart rate can point to dangerous arrhythmias. In addition to monitoring your vital signs after the surgery, the nurses will be checking the sensation and muscle strength in your extremities. If there are any unexpected abnormalities, your doctor will be notified.

As you wake up from the anesthesia, your pain may increase, and the nurses will provide you with pain medications appropriate to the level of pain you are experiencing. They will balance the reduction of your pain with minimizing the side effects of these medications, such as slowing down your breathing. Too much pain medication can, by decreasing the rate of your breathing, decrease the level of oxygen in your blood. Obviously, getting oxygen into your blood is vital to the body and your oxygen levels must be closely monitored. Fortunately, your brain has a system of stimulating and increasing your breathing rate anytime your blood oxygen levels fall.

PAIN — WHAT TO EXPECT

The intensity of pain that you will have after surgery depends on many factors. Some of these factors can be controlled, but others cannot be. The most important factor is obviously the type of surgery you had.

If you have undergone an epidural injection or another relatively simple and brief pain management procedure, postoperative recovery will most likely be straightforward, with a limited amount of pain. Some pain management specialists will not give you any sedating medications before an epidural injection. Others may choose to sedate you, to alleviate anxiety. If everything goes according to plan, you will be walking immediately after the procedure, and, in most cases, you will not be kept in the surgery center for more than one hour. If your doctor decides to sedate you before your procedure, the nurses will wait until you are no longer drowsy before sending you home. In most cases, no further pain medications will be required and you may resume your daily activities a few hours after the epidural injection. In fact, you can often return to work or even begin your physical therapy on the same day.

By comparison, a cervical discectomy and fusion will cause you to have more intense pain. Minimally invasive procedures are designed to have smaller incisions, which, in most cases, result in less pain, as do surgeries that are performed through the anterior approach, like anterior cervical fusion or anterior lumbar fusion. Surgeries that require a posterior approach and dissection through layers of muscle usually result in more pain.

Aches and Pains

If you pay close attention, you will notice that, every few minutes, you naturally change your position slightly when sitting or even when sleeping. This is a natural, protective phenomenon that prevents ulcerations and soft-tissue damage over the bony prominences of your body. During surgery, you will obviously not move at all. The longer the surgery, the greater the risk of developing ulcerations of your skin in vulnerable areas. The prominent areas of your bones will therefore have to be padded and protected. Still, when you wake up from your surgery, you may feel pain in body parts unrelated to the surgical site. This may be from pressure points or the position you were placed in during the surgery. Some surgical procedures, for example, require you to be placed on your abdomen for many hours. Pressure is usually placed on your pelvis and your chest. You may even experience chest pain after your surgery from this awkward position. This can sometimes be confused with a heart condition.

There are different tables on which your surgeon can perform your surgery. One elaborate type of table used during spine surgery is the Andrews table, which places you in a crawling position. Your legs are placed below the level of your abdomen, with your knees and hips in a ninety-degree flexed position. The advantage of this table is that it diverts blood to your legs and abdomen, which can decrease the amount of bleeding during surgery. It also arches your back, which can help your surgeon during the procedure. A post places pressure over each hip, and that can cause hip pain right after the surgery. This can be confused with the symptoms of persistent sciatica and radiculopathy (pain, numbness, or weakness due to a problem with the nerves). Even though this can be confusing, if your spine surgeon is experienced and knowledgeable, she will be able to differentiate between the two.

Methods of Pain Control

Your surgeon will have different ways of controlling your pain after surgery. The technique used will depend on the intensity of your pain and your medical history, as well as the extent of your surgery.

Local Anesthetics

You can surely remember that, at the dentist, you have been injected with medication to numb one area of your mouth. A similar type of medication that numbs your skin can be injected around your surgical wound. In most cases, the anesthetic Marcaine is used. The effect of this medication can last for many hours and can reduce your pain at least for that period of time after the surgery. Only the superficial layers of skin can be effectively numbed with this technique, but when it comes to pain, every little bit helps. Marcaine can effectively numb only small surgical sites like a microdecompression or a laminectomy incision. And, if this medication is injected into your bloodstream, the results can be catastrophic arrhythmias, which can be life-threatening. Fortunately, that is a rare complication.

Epidural Catheter

A pain-control technique that is somewhat controversial is the placement of an epidural catheter before surgery. This is similar to the epidural catheter that pregnant women receive before delivering their babies. Before the surgery, a catheter is placed next to the spine to slowly deliver a numbing medication to the lower part of the spinal cord after the surgery. The exact amount and concentration of this medication can be controlled to decrease pain around the lower back and the legs after surgery, while maintaining sensation and preserving your ability to move your legs.

This technique is controversial because it removes the protective nature of pain; the presence of excessive pain can indicate to your surgeon the presence of possible complications. Surgeons who decide to use an epidural catheter will place their patients in the intensive care unit to monitor them closely.

Oral Medications

If you are going to have an outpatient procedure like a microdiscectomy, the most common way to control your pain is by using oral pain medications. The most frequently used medications are hydrocodone-based, such as Vicodin or Norco. Tylenol #3 is another formulation, containing codeine instead of hydrocodone. All of these medications contain acetaminophen (Tylenol). Recently, other formulations have been developed that substitute an anti-inflammatory medication, such as ibuprofen, for acetaminophen.

You will find that you will need pain medication most on the day of surgery. As time goes by and your wound heals, your pain will decrease. It is very important to reduce your use of pain medications, since continued use can lead to tolerance and dependency, known as addiction.

Injectable Pain Medications

If you had more extensive surgery, your doctor may decide to admit you to the hospital for close monitoring as well as pain control. Here, your doctor will have many more choices in regard to pain medications. Injectable pain medications are much more potent and the dosage can be higher than that of oral pain medications that you can obtain from the pharmacy. Medications such as morphine, Dilaudid, or Demerol can be injected into the fat beneath your skin, within your muscle, or through an intravenous (IV) catheter directly into your blood vessels. The most rapid pain relief is provided when the medication is injected into a vein through your IV catheter, since this is the fastest route to your brain. It is also associated with the highest rate of complications. If too much pain medication is injected, it can cause your breathing to stop, which is the reason that intravenous injections of pain medication are usually done in an intensive care unit.

Patient-Controlled Analgesia (PCA) Pump

Since the most effective and rapid pain relief is achieved when the medication is injected into your vein, a machine has been devised called the patient-controlled analgesia pump (PCA). This type of pain control allows you to self-administer an effective dose of pain medication. You remain in the driver's seat in controlling your own pain, which, in most cases, results in greater patient satisfaction. The medication container is attached to a machine next to your bed. When you press a button, the machine releases a measured amount of the pain medication prescribed by your doctor, and it goes through the IV into your vein. The relief from your pain thus not only remains in your control; it is also almost instantaneous.

Your doctor will also determine the time allowed between each dose. If your doctor indicates that you should receive the medication every ten minutes, and you push the button seven minutes after you last pushed it, the machine will not release any medication. These are very important safeguards to avoid overmedication and unnecessary complications.

The PCA pump not only provides you with good pain control; it also eliminates the need to call a nurse each time you are having pain. Patients who are required to call the nursing staff commonly report dis-satisfaction with the length of time they have to wait to get pain medications. In most hospitals, it is fifteen to twenty minutes. This may be too long if you are in pain.

You can use the PCA pump up until the time you go home from the hospital. It is advisable, however, to stop the pump one day before your discharge and switch over to oral medications. This will allow you to test your ability to control your pain with oral medications, which will be the only mode of pain relief available at home.

YOUR SURGICAL WOUND

Your surgeon will use either staples or sutures to close the skin after surgery. Most surgeons will keep the staples or sutures in for about two weeks, at which time they will be removed in the office of your surgeon. An alternative technique for closing the site is absorbable sutures that are placed underneath the skin. In that case, most surgeons will choose to place special glue around the edges of your skin and cover it with medical tape called Steri-Strips. This is called a *subcuticular closure.* The sutures dissolve and the tape placed on your skin will eventually fall off.

Within five to seven days after the surgery, your body will naturally cover the surgical site with a layer of new skin; the incision will not be strong, however, after only seven days, and most surgeons agree that your wound should be kept clean and dry for at least ten days after the surgery. If you decide to take a shower after the surgery, you should make sure that your wound does not get wet. The technique recommended to care for your wound will depend upon the preference of your surgeon. In my practice, the surgical wound has a sterile dressing for ten days, at which time it can either be removed permanently or replaced by a new one, depending upon how well the wound has healed.

POSSIBLE COMPLICATIONS

Complications after surgery are common, but the most common complications are minor. Examples of minor complications include superficial wound infection, fever, or facial swelling. Catastrophic complications such as paralysis, deep infection, or nerve injury are uncommon but must be aggressively treated. An understanding of the possible complications may help you prevent a minor complication from developing into a major one.

Postsurgical Swelling

If your surgery is performed through the posterior approach, you will be lying on your abdomen, facing the floor, during the procedure. As a result, you will have swelling in your face and in all the areas that were hanging down toward the ground, since all the fluids in your body will be pulled downward by gravity. Facial swelling will resolve relatively quickly as your body excretes the excess fluid through your kidneys.

If you are a man, your testicles may swell to a massive size. In most cases, this should not cause alarm and the swelling will resolve spontaneously. If your surgery is a long one, your doctor will have inserted a Foley catheter to drain the urine from your bladder. This catheter will prevent collection of urine within your bladder and can help avoid complications. In the event that the testicles and penis swell, the catheter will continue to drain your urine until the swelling improves.

Fever

Most people who have surgery will have a few episodes of fever after the surgery. The source of fever after your surgery is most commonly the lungs. The most important and efficient way to prevent respiratory and lung infections is to take deep breaths during your recovery period. Walking after your surgery will result in deeper breathing than lying down and resting, and will reduce your chances of having respiratory infections and fever. Coughing is the most efficient way of expanding your lungs and getting rid of bacteria that can cause infections. Unfortunately, you may have pain at the surgical site with coughing or sneezing. Take deep breaths and walk if your surgeon has allowed you to do so after your surgery.

If you are in the hospital, your surgeon may order an *incentive spirometer*. This is a simple device that measures the depth of your breathing. It will encourage you to take deep breaths that can expand your lungs and prevent these common types of respiratory infections. You should use it every hour while in the hospital and should take it home with you, since these are disposable devices. Keep on using it until you have resumed your regular activities, which is usually about two weeks after your surgery.

Bladder or urinary tract infections (UTIs) may also cause fever after surgery. UTIs are much more common if a catheter was placed in your bladder before the procedure. It is very common to place a drainage tube in your bladder if the surgery is expected to take more than one hour. UTIs are much more common in women because of the relatively short distance between the environment and the bladder. In men, the penis places a longer distance between the environment and the bladder, which makes it more difficult for bacteria to travel into that organ. The detection of a UTI is done by testing a urine sample. If an infection is diagnosed, it can usually be cured with a few doses of antibiotics.

If you have fever, you are probably worried that you have a surgical wound infection. A surgical wound infection, however, is not the most common cause of a fever. As I have discussed, a respiratory or urinary infection is a much more common cause of fever in the early days after your surgery. In most cases, if a wound infection develops, it occurs about two weeks after the surgery. So, if you have fever within a few days after your surgery, don't be alarmed, but have your doctor keep a close eye on your wound. The first office visit after your surgery is mainly to check the site of the incision and make sure that an infection did not develop. Even though a wound infection is not the most common reason for fever after surgery, you should always be on the lookout for it, since a wound infection can turn a successful surgery into a complete failure.

Wound Infections

Without exception, your skin will be carefully prepared before your surgeon makes an incision. The science of skin preparation before surgery is precise. Many studies have examined how much bacterial contamination remains on the skin after it is prepared for surgery. The numbers of bacteria are low enough to make postoperative infections uncommon. Most surgeons will also administer some type of antibiotics before the surgery to reduce the risk of infection. Unfortunately, even with these precautions, the risk of postoperative infection is not totally eliminated, and special attention should be paid during the first three to four weeks after the surgery to insure that there is no infection developing in the area. It is important to inform your surgeon about any increasing pain at the site or any abnormal discharge from the wound. If there is an infection in your wound, the dressing can be visibly wet from the drainage. The severity of spinal wound infections can range from a superficial redness on the skin to a deep, paralyzing, catastrophic infection.

Natural Mechanisms That Fight Bacteria

Your body has many different mechanisms to combat bacteria. In fact, there is a constant battle between your body and bacteria, even without a surgical procedure. In the case of surgery, the most common path of entry is through the surgical wound. Bacteria can also enter the body through an area remote from the surgical wound, after which they are transported to the incision via the bloodstream. Upon entering the body, the bacteria will be attacked by antibodies, as well as by white blood cells. Your body has a library of antibodies that can fight different bacteria and viruses. If the bacteria are not killed quickly either by these natural antibodies, or by antibiotics, they will begin reproducing and cause an infection.

Risk Factors

If you have illnesses that decrease the strength of your skin or place you at a higher risk for an infection, special care must be taken during the days after the surgery. If you have diabetes, lupus, rheumatoid arthritis, or use steroids for any reason, chances of infection are higher and the healing process is slower.

Generally, as we have discussed, the bigger the incision and the longer the surgery, the higher your risk of infection. This is because bigger incisions and longer operating time increase the opportunities for bacteria to enter the surgical wound. In addition, the more the skin is retracted during surgery, the greater your risk of infection. Retraction of skin and soft tissues decreases the blood flow to the area. Since blood is the transportation vehicle for antibodies, white blood cells, and antibiotics, which combat bacteria, decreased blood flow can also increase the risk for infection. Aggressive retraction can also cause the death of local tissues, and the small amount of dead tissue can act as food for bacteria.

Additionally, if your surgeon inserts metallic implants during surgery, your risk of infection increases. Metallic implants act as housing for bacteria, which can take refuge from antibiotics and antibodies inside the implants. Because there is no blood flow through the metallic implants, the bacteria are protected in and around the crevices of the implants. Not only does the risk of infection increase with the placement of metallic implants, but also the severity of infections increases. Sometimes the infection will not resolve until the implants are removed.

What to Look For

If you develop an infection of your surgical wound, the most important thing is to inform your surgeon as soon as possible. The first question to be answered is whether the infection is deep-seated or limited to the superficial layers of the skin. Superficial infections of the skin and the underlying fat are common and can easily be treated with oral antibiotics. This scenario usually develops a few days after the surgery. You may have local pain at the surgical site, but no change in muscle strength or sensation will accompany superficial infections. You may or may not develop fever, since the infection is limited to a local area of skin.

In contrast, deep infections can have catastrophic consequences. They usually develop two weeks after the surgery. This timeline is consistent with the time that is required for the bacteria to replicate. The development of fever is much more common with deep infections. Drainage from the wound is frequently seen and will look like pus or a cloudy white fluid. The experience and judgment of your surgeon will play a large role in treating cases of infection.

Treatment

Depending on the physical examination and blood testing, your surgeon may decide to explore the wound in order to find out whether the infection is deep or superficial. Exploration of the wound will have its own set of risks, however. If there is no deep wound infection and only a superficial infection is detected, the infection can be introduced to the deeper layers, which can then worsen the infection. If a deep wound infection is detected, the wound will have to be irrigated with fluids to remove bacteria and devitalized tissue. This procedure is called *irrigation and debridement.*

If there are no metallic implants in the spine, there is a good chance that the infection will resolve with antibiotics, along with irrigation and debridement of the wound. If there are metallic implants within the wound and the surgery was performed recently, the usual recommendation is not to remove the implants initially. An infection that develops a few weeks after surgery has a better chance of resolving than an infection that develops months or years later. Infection that develops soon after surgery is called an *acute infection,* and an infection that develops months to years after surgery is called a *chronic infection.* Your surgeon may irrigate and debride your infected wound several times. If, after several attempts, your infection does not resolve, she may consider removing the metallic implants. Depending upon the reason that the implants were first inserted, she may or may not be able to remove them. In cases of chronic infection, your surgeon is more likely to remove the metallic implants, since the bones have fused and healed by then.

One interesting technique for combating a surgical wound infection is to mix antibiotic powder with cement powder. The powder mix is then turned into liquid surgical cement and made into small balls, which harden in a few minutes and are then placed in the infected wound. The antibiotic within the cement is slowly released over a period of six weeks. The concentration of antibiotics released in the wound is extremely high, compared with other delivery methods such as intravenous or oral administration. When the infection is resolved and the antibiotics are completely released from the cement balls, the cement can either be removed or left within the wound. Most spine surgeons are familiar with this technique.

Deep Venous Thrombosis (DVT) and Pulmonary Embolism (PE)

Deep venous thrombosis (DVT) means the formation of a blood clot, which most commonly develops in the legs. Most blood clots will stay in the deep veins of your legs. But sometimes they can loosen and travel to your heart or lung. A blood clot that moves to your heart or lung is called a *pulmonary embolism* (PE). A DVT is not dangerous unless it turns into a PE.

A DVT can develop in your legs in many different situations, usually when you are immobile for an extended period, as, for example, during a long airplane flight, prolonged bed rest, or surgery. During short surgical procedures, the danger of developing a DVT is low and it is not always necessary to take steps to prevent one. The risk becomes significant, however, during surgical procedures that are longer than one or two hours. To help avert the risk of DVT, a machine called a *sequential compression device* can be used during surgery. It pushes on your calves to assist in circulating blood toward your heart. Most hospitals use these devices routinely for spine surgery.

Preventing blood clots after the surgery should be an ongoing concern for you and your doctor. The best way to prevent DVTs is to walk. The act of walking requires complex and forceful muscle contractions, which push on the blood vessels that pump the blood away from the legs and toward the heart. This prevents the blood from remaining stagnant in the vessels and thwarts the development of DVTs. If your doctor has instructed you to avoid walking, or you have stopped walking due to pain, you should take other precautions to avoid DVTs in your legs. One other way to reduce your risk of developing a DVT is to keep your legs elevated. Another is to periodically move your feet toward your head (flex them). This requires muscle contractions of your calf muscles which will result in increased blood circulation toward your heart.

The most common complaint that you will have if there is a DVT in your legs is pain in your calves. Unfortunately, this can be confusing if you are suffering from a herniated lumbar disc or sciatica, since the pain from these conditions can mimic the pain of a DVT. You may also develop swelling in your leg because of a blood clot. Most doctors who suspect the presence of a DVT will request an ultrasound of the legs. In most cases, the detection of a DVT is relatively easy and it can be treated with blood-thinning medications. Unfortunately, however, you will not be able to take these medications for at least a few days after your surgery. Taking blood-thinning medications too soon after your surgery can result in dangerous bleeding in your spine. An alternative treatment is the placement of a small filter in a large vein called the *vena cava*. This vein delivers the blood from your legs back to the heart. If a blood clot dislodges from your legs and moves toward the heart, it will be caught by the filter. This will prevent a life-threatening blockage of the heart and lung vessels.

WALKING AFTER SURGERY

With recent advancements in spine surgery and the development of quality implants, it would be unusual for your surgeon to instruct you to avoid walking after the surgery. In most cases, your surgeon will urge you to begin walking as soon as your pain permits you to do so. Many of the difficulties that you may have after the operation will resolve more quickly if you begin walking soon after your surgery. As we discussed, most people will have a fever after the surgery from the anesthesia and the fact that their lungs are not fully expanded. Walking causes you to take deep breaths, which inflates the lungs and clears any bacteria that may be sitting deep within them. This can resolve any fever that you may have.

You will most likely have difficulties moving your bowels after your surgery, which is the result of the anesthesia. Walking and resuming your regular activities will also lead to a faster resumption of intestinal activity. Eradicating constipation after the surgery is very important and can reduce your pain substantially. Many times, patients complain of back pain that is actually the result of constipation, and they find that it resolves after a bowel movement.

HELP AT HOME AFTER YOUR SURGERY

What kind of help will you need at home after your surgery? This will depend upon your age and your physical ability, as well as your motivation before the surgery. The younger you are, the better your ability will be to physically cope with the surgery. No matter what your age, though, it is very important for you to maintain good family support and make all the preparations necessary before the surgery. Stairs will be difficult to negotiate after the procedure, and if you live in a multilevel house or apartment building, try to stay on a lower floor. Arrangements can be made before the surgery for a hospital bed to be provided when you come home. Going to the bathroom may be difficult and a bedside commode may resolve that issue. Shower chairs as well as a railing within your shower will help you return to your lifestyle more quickly. Other aids that you may think about are walkers, as well as instruments to pick up objects from the floor without the need to bend. Those can be obtained from medical supply stores. Many of these items may be covered by your health insurance; be sure to check well before the surgery.

If your surgery is complex, your surgeon may arrange for a visiting nurse to insure that no complications are missed during your postoperative recovery time. Home aid is another service that may be available in your area. Social services can be provided to you for preparation of meals as well as general cleaning duties. Inquire with your insurance company as well as the office of your surgeon regarding these services well before the operation to avoid confusion afterward.

POSTSURGICAL THERAPY

Your spine surgeon will make recommendations for therapy depending on the type of surgery you had. In most cases it will be difficult for you to start therapy immediately after the surgery. It is a good idea to allow your wounds to heal before beginning any type of therapy. Even massage therapy, which is relatively passive, can complicate your wound-healing process and is not suggested immediately after your operation. Spinal fusion procedures require that therapy be delayed for at least one to two months, since excessive range of motion can delay bony fusion as well as recovery. The one type of therapy that can be helpful right after surgery is ambulation training, which you can do with a physical therapist. Since there is such a variation in the timeline for beginning therapy after your surgery, it is best to discuss this specific issue with the surgeon who has actually performed the operation.

*   *   *

With luck, you have not had any of the complications I've described and your recovery is going smoothly. Even if you have had some difficulty, knowledge is your best tool in bouncing back quickly. Once you are up on your feet and back to your usual routine, it's time to plan for a healthy back for life, and that's just what we'll do in the book's next section. We'll look at how you can prevent future back problems by keeping your back strong and using nutrition and ergonomics in optimal ways.

PART THREE

A Healthy Back for Life

INTRODUCTION

It's a new you—healthy, strong, and motivated to stay that way. Hopefully you have taken action and resolved your back pain through the best possible approach for your condition. Now what can you do to maintain spinal health?

Chapter 7 gives you ideas and techniques on how to prevent further back problems. You will receive tips on proper posture regarding walking, standing, sitting, and sleeping. Moreover, exercise guidelines and benefits will be discussed; you might even decide to become "addicted to exercise" after reading this part of *Back Surgery: Is It Right for You?* Nutrition is also briefly considered because it is such an integral part of health maintenance.

Lastly, Chapter 8 tackles something that too many sources like to avoid—the connection between back pain and psychology. There is a good chance that someone who has experienced significant back pain has also experienced some level of depression. Is one condition causing the other, or exacerbating the other? If this sounds like something to which you are vulnerable, are you working with a practitioner who is understanding of the connection? Before we close this book, let's make sure we are headed as much toward a healthy state of mind as we are toward a healthy state of body. Only then can we finally say that you're "back" in action and ready for a new day.

7

Preventing Future Back Problems

Whether you have already had surgery, or you are attempting to avoid surgery altogether, it is essential that you keep your back strong and healthy. I hope this chapter will help you in this endeavor! We will begin the chapter with an examination of the importance of posture and will move toward a discussion of exercises that will keep your back strong, flexible, and resistant to injury and pain.

IMPROVING YOUR POSTURE

Believe it or not, posture is one of your strongest weapons in the fight to protect your back. That's because your spine has been designed to have several curves in it, each of which balances the other. There is a relatively large curve in your midback, which balances two smaller curves in your neck and lower back. The relationship of all these curves results in a relatively straight posture, which aligns your neck precisely over your pelvis. When your posture is correct, the muscles in and around your spine do not have to do much work in maintaining a balanced position. If your posture is off balance, some of the muscles have to work constantly to bring your posture into correct alignment. This requires energy and, over a long period of time, can cause fatigue and pain. It is possible to measure muscle activity in the laboratory, and it has been shown that the forces in and around the spinal column are lowest when the posture is balanced and without movement.

Feet

Good posture begins in your feet. Feet that are rotated inward or out-ward can cause changes in your gait, which can in turn cause further pressure and strain on the muscles of your back. Relieving an abnormal position of your feet with special shoes or orthotics can minimize the pressure placed on the spine. Unfortunately, most spine surgeons will not pay much attention to your feet in searching for the cause of your back pain. Most will search for structural abnormalities in your spinal column before looking at other causes, such as unusual foot placement or abnormal foot structure.

The specialists who are most concerned with the posture of the feet are *podiatrists*. Their primary education centers on the feet and they also have special training in the fabrication of shoe inserts to correct any mis-alignment of your feet. These misalignments can come about for many reasons, including a birth defect or a fracture that healed abnormally.

Legs

A related issue is the common condition in which the legs are different lengths. It is not unusual to have one leg longer than the other, but in most cases this discrepancy is small and not noticeable. Unfortunately, if this discrepancy is subtle, it is likely to have been there silently for many years and to have gone undetected. As the years go by, the effects of this condition will often begin to emerge in the form of hip and back pain. Only a very careful search will detect this subtle abnormality, which can bring your pelvis out of balance and tilt it to the side. This in turn will cause your spine to tilt, and the effects can be seen all the way up to your neck.

If the discrepancy in the length of your legs is more than one inch, you should consider a visit to your foot specialist to get special shoe inserts to elevate the shorter leg. If the discrepancy is small—up to one or two inches—a shoe insert can correct the problem while the insert remains undetectable within your shoe.

A more pronounced discrepancy in the length of the lower extremi-ties is easily detectable, and can result in significant postural abnormal-ities such as scoliosis. This, and other deformities caused by a difference in the length of the lower extremities, can slowly worsen, leading to severe arthritis and pain in adulthood. If the leg discrepancy is large, you will need special shoes that are custom-made and have a heel of the appropriate height for each leg. The compensations built into these shoes are more difficult to hide, and you will be limited in the type of shoes you can wear. In most cases, you should not seek treatment for the discrepancy in the length of your legs from your spine surgeon. Once the condition is detected, you should see a podiatrist for appropriate treatment, which should be relatively simple to arrange.

Shoulders, Chest, and Pelvis

Another element in good posture is your shoulders being pushed backward and your chest pushed forward. You can see an exaggeration of this type of posture in military trainees. Remember that your pelvis is the most important segment of your body in keeping a good posture. Your pelvis should be tilted backward. If you do all of this correctly, your neck will be positioned between your shoulder blades and centered directly over your pelvis. This will place the least amount of pressure over the structures of your spine, which will remain pain-free and healthy.

Hamstrings

The position of your pelvis is controlled by the hamstring muscles, in the back of your legs. The hamstring muscles attach to the pelvis and to the knee. If your hamstring muscles are tight, your pelvis will be pulled into a forward-flexed posture. This, in turn, will place your spine in an unfavorable position, leading to back pain. It will also keep your neck moving in a forward direction, which will cause your back to assume a hump in its midregion. Your chest will then move backward, and your entire posture will fall out of alignment.

For this reason, you will hear many athletic trainers emphasizing the need to stretch your hamstrings. There are several different ways to stretch your hamstring muscles. One simple technique is to stand erect and to bend forward slowly in an attempt to touch your toes. This will stretch your hamstrings, but will also place pressure on your spine. Performing this type of exercise will be difficult if you have back problems. You should attempt to do this slowly, increasing flexibility over time. Another technique for stretching your hamstrings is to lie on the floor while placing your legs on the wall. You must remember to keep your pelvis flat on the floor. This will maintain your spine in a straight position while stretching your hamstrings.

The best way to stretch your hamstrings requires the help of another person. A personal trainer will have you lie flat on the floor. One of his hands will keep your pelvis flat on the floor. The trainer will use one of his legs to place pressure over the leg that is not being stretched. He will then bring the other leg straight up, keeping the knee extended. Your spine will remain flat and the muscles free of stress. This will produce the maximum amount of stretch for your hamstrings. Your trainer will be able to feel how tight your hamstrings really are and can guide you in this process.

Changing Your Position Often

Maintaining good posture does not mean staying in the same position at all times. Periodic change in the position in which you are standing or sitting is important and makes sense. Even when you maintain good posture, there will be some muscle activity holding your position. Varying this position will change the muscles that are maintaining your posture, thereby shifting the workload among different muscle groups. This can help avoid fatigue and injury to the muscles and the structures of your back.

If you are required to sit or stand for more than a short period of time, try leaning against an object or giving support to your arms. The help that you get from a wall or table can substantially decrease the strain on your muscles. For example, if you are washing dishes or working at a machine in a factory, change the position of your foot by placing it on a footstool and get support by putting your arms on a nearby table. If you work as a security officer, alternate placing your weight on the other leg every few minutes.

In general, "standing tall" is the term used by many physical therapists in order to summarize all the factors that I mentioned to you just now. It means pulling in your stomach and buttocks while getting into a straight-line posture. If your posture is maintained correctly, the least amount of pressure will be placed on the structures of your spine. Maintenance of good posture, however, is important not only when you are standing still, but when you are sitting, lying down, or lifting.

SITTING

It is much more common to be sitting for extended periods than standing. Most jobs that require maintaining a stationary position for extended periods involve sitting. The subject of ergonomic workstation modification is extremely important. Chronic back pain can lead to disability and loss of time from work, along with the dissatisfaction of employees. A relatively small investment by the employer can result in increased productivity, and decreased need for breaks by their employees, which can dramatically increase the bottom line for the company. A happy employee is unlikely to change jobs, which can also eliminate the need for rehiring and retraining. Ergonomic workstation restructuring should not be regarded as an unnecessary cost, but rather as a fruitful investment.

An Ergonomic Chair

If you are sitting on a chair during an eight-hour shift, you should consider an ergonomic chair that will reduce the stress placed on your back. A good chair will support the curves in your back. Straightening of the normal lumbar arch can have consequences for your neck, as well as your mid- and lower back, leading to fatigue and muscle spasms after ten to fifteen minutes of continuous sitting. Most ergonomic chairs will have a lumbar curve support that maintains the arch in your lower back. The more expensive models will even have an adjustable curve support for your lower back. Most ergonomic chairs will also have a relatively tall back support that extends beyond your midback.

The second factor in choosing the correct chair is the height adjustment. The chair should adjust to a height that matches the desk you are working on. If the chair is too low, it will result in your neck being extended and your arms being higher than they should be, preventing them from supporting your body weight. If the chair is too high, it will cause your neck to flex excessively and your wrists to extend. This can cause tendonitis and wrist pain, along with neck pain and unnecessary strain to your back. The proper height will decrease pressure on your wrists as you are typing or writing. Since it is difficult to predict the exact level of your desk, it is much easier to have a chair with an adjustable height. Most ergonomic chairs will have hydraulic pumps that can easily adjust the height of the chair.

The armrests of the chair are also very important. The more expensive chairs will allow you to adjust their height. You should be able to rest your elbows on the armrests, which will in turn decrease the stress placed on your spine. If the armrests are too short, your arms will not reach them, rendering them useless. If they are too high, they will cause your arms and shoulders to fan out to reach those heights. They should be adjustable so that you can comfortably use them.

You will sink into a chair with a seat that is too soft, which is not good for your posture. A chair that you can sink into will transfer the pressure to your lower back, and cause a curved and slouchy posture. A cushion seat that is too firm may cause pressure sores over the bony prominences of your pelvis. Test the seat cushion before buying the chair, since the desired firmness is a personal feel that is different for each person. It is similar to buying a bed!

The edge of the seat should be rounded, in order to avoid pressure on your hamstring muscles. As I have already mentioned, maintaining flexibility in the hamstring muscles is very important to keeping an appropriate pelvic tilt. If the edge of the seat is not rounded, it may cause muscle irritation, which can result in spasm and pain.

Some companies have realized that an ergonomic chair should have multiple adjustments to conform to the individual needs of each person. The difference between very tall and short people may be so great that one chair will not fit everyone. For that reason, companies have surfaced that will manufacture custom-made ergonomic chairs that are tailored to your individual needs. Unfortunately, the price for such a chair is usually higher than for a ready-made chair that you can buy in most stores.

Other Elements of Your Ergonomic Workstation

It is not only the chair that should be ergonomically positioned, although that is obviously the most important aspect of an ergonomic workstation. You can decrease tension in your spine by allowing your legs to rest comfortably on a footrest. Your computer station and monitor should be maintained at the level of your eyes to avoid excessive flexion or extension of your neck. You should avoid placing your monitor and keyboard to the side, even though it may be more practical to do so, in order to make more space on your desk. The consequences of pain and stiffness will not be worth the added space. By placing the keyboard and monitor to the side, you will have to keep either your lower back or your neck and arms in a twisted position. In either case, you are sure to suffer from the consequences of incorrect posture. To make more room on your desk, try installing a keyboard drawer instead. It will rest under your table and it can be rolled away when not in use. There are also adjustable monitor holders that are commercially available and will attach to almost any desk.

Headphones

If you are using the phone more than just occasionally, headphones are an ideal solution. Without the headphones, you are likely to hold the phone between your shoulder and your ear. Most people will just use one side of the head, which will only worsen the problem. You may use a shoulder rest for your phone, but unfortunately these are not ideal. Even with a shoulder rest on your telephone, you can still find yourself bending your neck to hold the phone to your ear, which can cause unnecessary strain to your neck muscles. So the best option still remains the headphones.

DRIVING

Your posture matters when you are driving a car, too. You can use most of the principles that I have already mentioned and apply them to your posture when you are sitting in a car. One factor that will work against you is the constant shaking and vibration that your spine is exposed to when driving. A healthy spine can tolerate the vibrations and the small impact that each bump causes to the spine, but if you suffer from back pain, you will surely have noticed that driving for more than twenty minutes causes a flare-up in your pain. Back-pain sufferers will usually report more pain to their spine specialist after driving to the office. It is the car ride itself that causes this increased pain and can confuse the physician and the patient. Traveling in an airplane or on a motorcycle can have similar effects.

If you are suffering from mechanical back pain, you will surely notice that your pain increases when you sit for an extended period. This is because the pressure on your discs is the greatest when you sit, and it decreases when you stand or lie down. The maximum pressure on the discs in your back occurs when you are sitting at a 90-degree angle. Fortunately, when you're sitting in a car or an airplane, you can decrease the pressure on the discs in your spine by bringing your seat to a reclining position. Lowering your seat to a 110-degree angle will markedly decrease the pressure on your discs, which in turn will lessen the pain.

SLEEPING

Although you may never have thought about it, your posture when you sleep is vital, too. Maintaining the correct alignment of the curvature of your spine can help avoid unnecessary strain on the muscles in your back and decrease the stress and pressure on the discs of your spine. Many sources will attempt to give you advice on which position to use when sleeping. Unfortunately, the position in which you choose to sleep will not always be under your control and you will surely find yourself sleeping in a different position when you wake up. For this reason, suggestions regarding specific sleeping positions are not useful. One thing you do have control over, however, is your mattress.

It is generally accepted among doctors that a firm mattress is preferable to a soft mattress, which will not support the necessary curves of your back and will allow the midportion of your body to fall deep into the mattress. You should keep in mind that a firm mattress will cause you some body aches if you sleep mostly on your side. A very firm mattress will not conform to the natural curvature of your hips and your rib cage when you sleep on your side. The newer model high-quality mattresses will incorporate a very firm type of mattress with a soft cushion top. This combines the best of two worlds, giving you the sensation of a soft mattress with a firm deeper structure.

Choosing your mattress can be extremely difficult. Have you tried to find the same model and make of a mattress in two different stores? This is usually an impossible task. Most mattress stores sell the same mattress under a different name. This is because most retail stores have a low-price guarantee if you find the same mattress at a lower price. By changing the name of the mattress, this price war is avoided and you, the consumer, remain in the dark as to the true price of your mattress.

Unfortunately, there are no clear guidelines in choosing the right mattress. Fortunately, some mattress stores do allow you to exchange your mattress one or two weeks after buying it if you find it to be uncomfortable. Even though those stores may sell you a mattress at a higher price, having the choice of exchanging a mattress is surely better than blindly buying a firm mattress that was recommended by your spine specialist. If your mattress is uncomfortable and you no longer have the option of exchanging your mattress, another option is to place a mattress pad below your sheet and over your mattress. In this way, you can fine-tune the firmness of your mattress.

LIFTING

Using a proper lifting technique is one way to protect your spine. Most people who have suffered from a lumbar disc herniation report that the disc herniation occurred when they were lifting something. The greatest pressures are exerted on the spine when you are bending forward while attempting to lift or carry an object that you are holding away from your body. Furthermore, when you bend your back to lift an object, the muscles in your lower back are stretched, which makes them vulnerable to injury. If you lift the same object while keeping your back straight, the pressures within the discs don't increase nearly as much. And, if you keep the object as close to your body as possible, you will decrease the stress placed on your muscles. Instead of bending your back, rely on your leg muscles. The muscles in your legs are extremely strong and were designed for this task.

Many athletes, as well as work injury prevention experts, advocate using a lumbar corset when performing lifting activities. The use of a lumbar corset increases abdominal pressure and, in theory, will provide further support to your back. This is important when you are required to lift or push an object. The use of a lumbar brace also helps you to remember to maintain good posture and can remind you of a back injury if you have one. Studies have not conclusively shown, however, that wearing a lumbar corset can actually decrease the chance of injury to your back. Controversy also exists about whether a lumbar corset may even decondition the back muscles, causing them to lose strength and the ability to cope with sudden stresses to the spine. Even though there is no clear evidence that a lumbar support corset prevents injuries, many employers of people who are required to perform heavy lifting still recommend their use in an attempt to minimize the chances of injury.

STRENGTHENING YOUR BODY

It is important to keep the back muscles stretched, flexible, and strong. The stronger these muscles, the more they can support the spinal column and cope with everyday tasks without getting injured. Maintaining good posture will keep your lower back muscles ready for unexpected stresses, such as lifting a heavy object. This is the difference between the experience of an athlete who lifts heavy weights and the experience of the ordinary person; because of their strength training, athletes have great posture. The other reason that athletes don't get injured with heavy lifting is that they anticipate the weight of the object and their brain recruits all the necessary muscles before the lifting actually occurs. Most injuries occur when you don't expect the object to be as heavy as it actually is and you exceed the weight your back muscles can tolerate.

Another common cause of injury in the nonathletic person is sudden, unexpected twisting, which results in the tearing of muscles that are not trained and are deconditioned. By performing strength exercises, you increase the weight that your muscles can lift. And by performing endurance exercises, you increase the time that your muscles can maintain the force to support that weight. These elements of exercise will be discussed shortly.

What about support to your spine from the front of your body? Surely you have seen competitive athletes lifting heavy weights. They all wear strong abdominal belts. These belts support the abdominal muscles to increase the pressure within the abdomen. This increased pressure supports the spinal column from the front. Well-toned abdominal muscles—such as the *rectus abdominis,* commonly referred to as the "six-pack"—will increase the pressure within your abdomen, which will in turn support your spine, like the weight lifter's abdominal belt. Poorly toned abdominal muscles, by contrast, will allow your abdominal contents to push forward. This is the so-called "beer belly." Since the abdominal contents are allowed to push out and forward, more of your body weight is placed in front of your spine, which in turn causes your spine to sway forward. Your posture assumes a forward position that will place further stress on your spinal column.

Don't forget to put exercises to strengthen your abdominal muscles into your exercise routine. Maintaining strong abdominal muscles is just as important as keeping your back muscles strong.

Exercise Guidelines

Guidelines have been established by the American Academy of Orthopaedic Surgeons with regard to the need for exercise in preventing or reducing back pain. Most people should exercise three to four days a week for at least twenty minutes to maintain healthy posture and strong muscles, as well as flexibility. This is also a good way to maintain healthy joints.

You might be wondering why a twenty-minute minimum of exercise is required. It takes twenty minutes of aerobic activity to start reaping health benefits. The American College of Sports Medicine defines aerobic exercise as any activity that uses large muscle groups, is maintained continuously, and is rhythmic in nature. Some examples of aerobic exercise include jogging, swimming, dancing, biking, cross-country skiing, in-line skating, jumping rope, and stair climbing. There are several different techniques you can use to insure that you are performing aerobic exercise. The simplest is to measure your heart rate during the aerobic exercise. If your heart rate is between 60 and 90 percent of your maximal heart rate, then you are performing an aerobic exercise. Your maximal heart rate can be calculated by subtracting your age from the number 220.

The Three Aspects of Muscle Training

In regard to muscle training, exercise has three different aspects. One aspect is strength training, the second is endurance training, and the last is flexibility training. Depending on the type of exercise that you do, you may benefit unevenly with regard to strength, endurance, and flexibility. Each type of exercise provides your back with a different tool in preventing and recovering from injury or surgery. Building strength means being able to lift heavier weights without injuring your back. Endurance refers to the ability to have a prolonged muscle contraction when performing a task. This means maintaining a relatively stressful position, as, for example, when you are washing dishes in a flexed posture. It is generally accepted that strength training is important for females and endurance training is important for males. Stretching, on the other hand, prepares the muscles, tendons, and ligaments to accept sudden changes in position and provides the flexibility to put your spine in a wider range of motion.

The Benefits of Exercise

Exercise benefits almost every part of your body. Let's look at some of the specific ways your health will improve with exercise.

Your Bones and Muscles

Exercise prevents and can even reverse osteoporosis. Active strength training stresses the bones, as do impact aerobic exercises such as jumping rope. This type of exercise stimulates bone metabolism and increases the mineral content of your bones, resulting in stronger bones. Exercise also builds stronger muscles, which act as a protective cover to the bones, reducing the risk of fractures in the elderly.

From Cholesterol to Diabetes

Exercise not only improves your musculoskeletal health; it also benefits your internal organs. Exercise has been shown to reduce cholesterol and may be even more effective than medication in this regard. Most physicians who prescribe medication to reduce cholesterol also prescribe an exercise program. Exercise can also stabilize and lower both the systolic and diastolic values of your blood pressure, which reduces your risk of a stroke or heart attack. In addition, exercise has been shown to reduce the risk of Alzheimer's and dementia in the elderly.

If you are diabetic, your glucose tolerance will improve with exercise. In fact, exercise can even prevent adult-onset diabetes. If you are overweight and just developed diabetes, you can reverse and normalize your blood sugar levels by reducing your weight with exercise, which also improves and increases metabolic activity. Muscles require energy to survive, and increased muscle mass in your body will increase your energy requirements even at rest. Once you build muscles, they will continue to burn calories even when you are resting. Think of muscle building as an investment in maintaining a healthy and strong back, along with a lower weight, which results in a visually pleasing body.

Increased Libido

Another health benefit of exercise is an increase in your sexual desire, also called libido, which may affect your relationships in a positive manner. Women and men who exercise routinely report improved sex life and increased satisfaction from their relationship. People who exercise routinely are aroused to sexual stimulation faster and more intensely. This may be a result of the increased self-esteem that exercise brings or of increased stamina, since intense and prolonged sexual activity requires strong muscles with endurance. Furthermore, sexual activity itself can cause back injury, which can be prevented by muscular strength and endurance training.

Decreased Depression

In addition to all its other benefits, exercise is known to reduce stress, elevate your spirit, and even fight the symptoms of depression. It is well known that depression and back pain are closely linked. If, in fact, exercise does reduce the symptoms of depression, it can directly and indirectly fight back pain and its disabling symptoms. The mechanism that exercise uses to fight depression may be related to the release of chemicals known as *endorphins* in your body. Endorphins are naturally produced by the pituitary gland in the brain, in response to certain stimuli. They are very similar to opioids like morphine and even attach to the same receptors in the body. Endorphins produce a pleasing feeling of well-being. This is one way that your body signals to you to repeat behavior that results in a pleasurable outcome, such as eating, sexual activity, drug use, and even seeing a loved one. When exercising, muscles that work hard release chemicals that cause your blood to become slightly acidic. This is called *acidosis*. Acidosis, caused by lactic acid, causes the pituitary gland (in your brain) to release endorphins.

"Addiction" to Exercise

Over the long term, you can develop an addiction to exercise, since, as we have just seen, each time you exercise, a bolus of endorphins is released into your bloodstream. Many athletes do describe their behavior with regard to exercise as an addiction. These athletes also describe symptoms of depression when they stop exercising. Unfortunately, this addiction does not develop quickly, and if you are just starting to exercise, you are likely to experience pain from deconditioned muscles and lack of endurance, instead of euphoria. The development of endurance, strength, and flexibility requires time, effort, and discipline. You must be persistent in order to be able to exercise for any significant length of time and develop this good type of addiction. If you have just started exercising, don't expect to be able to exercise strenuously, or feel the rush of endorphins in your body within the first or second session. With discipline and persistence, however, you will experience the many benefits that exercise can bring to your body, your spine, and your life.

Other health benefits of exercise are still surfacing, but it is generally accepted that the human body was not designed for a sedentary lifestyle, to which most people today are accustomed. As our lives have evolved over the past thousands of years, so have our daily habits. Our bodies were designed to hunt for our food, walk to our destinations, and perform strenuous activities throughout the day. Today, we attain food without any significant effort. Our preferred mode of transportation is the automobile. And most strenuous activities are performed by technologically advanced machines. As a result, some people now exercise in a gym to make up for our "unnaturally" sedentary lifestyle. Keep in mind that as our bodies evolve, so do the ailments that affect our spines. Sedentary lifestyle may not affect the rate of congenital conditions from which our spines suffer, but the incidence of common back strains and sprains is certainly higher.

If you attempt to enter into an exercise program that requires heavy lifting for extended periods, you may be exposing your back to stress that it is not accustomed to. This, by itself, can cause injury. Performing controlled types of exercise, on the other hand, will slowly lead to strength and endurance without causing any further injury. No matter what exercise you decide to do, you should always remember to do it in a controlled manner, slowly increasing the duration of the exercise as well as the amount of weight you lift during the exercise. For example, you may decide to start swimming, and at first you may be able to swim for five minutes. If you initially attempt to perform that exercise for twenty minutes, you will find yourself sore, with recurrent back pain that may linger for more than two weeks. In contrast, if you slowly work your way up to twenty minutes of swimming, you may find that pain will be nonexistent, and if it was present before the exercise, it will slowly improve.

Swimming is regarded as the best exercise for your back. It decreases the amount of stress to your back because it will not allow you to make sudden movements even if you try. It also allows you to exercise your back as you propel through the water. Running, by contrast, may not be as beneficial to you if you suffer from chronic back pain. No studies have conclusively shown that running aggravates back injury, but many spine surgeons have reservations about running when it comes to patients with chronic back pain. Since it has not been conclusively shown that running is an exercise that should not be performed, the best advice is to increase the intensity and duration of this activity slowly, as you would with any exercise.

NUTRITION AND WEIGHT CONTROL

There are several reasons that nutrition is key in preventing problems with your back. First, the intake of nutrients such as calcium and vitamin D is important for bone strength; second, good nutrition helps you maintain optimal weight to decrease stress on the structures of the spine; and finally, new studies have shown a correlation between high cholesterol and degenerative disc disease.

As we grow into adulthood, developing in size and shape, our bones slowly accumulate calcium to maintain strength. Our intake of calcium also increases bone density. The accumulation of calcium is closely regulated by many factors, one of which is vitamin D. During the second half of our lives, our bodies are depleted of calcium and, as we reach the age of sixty and beyond, we tend to lose calcium rapidly from our bones, which can place us at higher risk for insufficiency fractures of the hip and wrist, as well as compression fractures of the spine. If you are a thin, elderly white woman, you are at the highest risk of developing this type of fracture. In order to avoid such fractures when you are older, you must start consuming vitamin D and calcium early on in life. Heavy exercise, such as impact aerobics, increases the stress on your bones, thereby stimulating the deposit of calcium in your bones—also called *mineralization*—which strengthens them.

Being overweight can be detrimental to your back. Imagine carrying a backpack weighing thirty pounds on your back throughout the day. How about carrying a grocery bag weighing thirty pounds for one hour? You can easily see that being overweight places stress on your joints as well as your bones. It will make you sluggish and can even prevent you from performing exercise. The excess weight can cause you to enter a vicious cycle of inactivity and increased weight. The excess weight will not only strain your back, but will also tax your heart, kidneys, and vascular system. Furthermore, it places stress on your hips, knees, and ankles, which can lead to early arthritis and further inactivity from the arthritis itself. And excess weight can cause diabetes, kidney failure, and hypertension. Maintaining your weight in the normal range is important to almost every system in your body, including your psychological health.

If you just started a diet and exercise program, you have undoubt-edly noticed that the most difficult period is the first two or three weeks. You will feel very tired and develop soreness in almost every muscle that you use. Remember, there will be a big reward: a leaner body that is more functional and more visually appealing.

*   *   *

We've just taken a look at some of the many ways you can strengthen your back and prevent back problems: by improving your posture when standing, sitting, lifting, and even sleeping; by exercising; and by getting proper nutrition and shedding excess pounds. There is another element, however, that can help you overcome back problems: your psychological outlook. We'll examine that important factor in the next chapter.

8

Psychology and Back Pain

"It's all in your head." Believe it or not, that still might be the comment you hear from a very few back surgeons, or, more likely, it could be your own nagging thought about your nagging pain. Or how about, "It's mind over matter; you can will away your back pain." Both of these scenarios are woefully lacking and rarely accurate. Your mind can, however, play an essential role in both your pain and your recovery, so it's important to take a look at the psychological issues that might be part of the picture.

Before you can begin to understand the significance of psychology as it relates to back pain, we must establish that the words "all" and "none" do not apply to this subject. Keep in mind that every situation is different and that the psychological and physical aspects of your pain are related in a unique way in your case. If you are considering a doctor who has said that the source of all pain is the same and there is one treatment for all back problems, think twice about your choice.

OLD THEORIES PERSIST

In your quest to find answers to your questions, you will encounter books and articles that attempt to explain the source of all your pain on the basis of one theory alone. Some writers suggest, for example, that the cause of all back pain is psychological, even in the presence of structural or anatomical abnormalities. These authors claim that tension, depression, stress, or other psychological conditions are the sole cause of back pain. They argue that the treatment of the psychological condition will resolve your back pain, and that, if your back pain persists, it simply indicates that the psychological condition was treated inappropriately. This explanation is neither realistic nor responsible.

"Mind over Pain"

The idea of mind over pain is not new. It was a philosophy long before sophisticated medical imaging was ever on the scene. Fifty years ago, the diagnosis of a back condition was guesswork at best, and the treatment for it was even more elusive. At that time, the term "back pain" was an actual diagnosis. Today, we know it to be just a symptom of other back conditions. Since the diagnosis and treatment of back pain were so difficult, the treatment was usually unsuccessful. Many patients continued to suffer from back pain for unexplained reasons. Some medical professionals who were trained then still believe that the cause of back pain is mostly psychological.

Tension myositis syndrome (TMS) is one example of this type of psychologically oriented theory. It claims that the cause of back pain is not structural, but is rather related to the inflammation of muscles due to circulatory changes. The theory suggests that these circulatory changes result from the constriction of blood vessels, which in turn deprive the muscles of blood. Proponents of the TMS theory believe that tension and stress cause all these problems, which are in turn the root of all back pain. The theory does not recognize structural abnormalities, such as herniated discs, degenerative discs, spondylolisthesis, not to mention cancer or scoliosis, as possible causes of back pain. This theory may explain some cases of back pain, but it is probably a very small percentage of all cases. Furthermore, the theory can't be proven by any diagnostic study offered by today's advanced medicine.

"Matter Alone Matters"

There are many surgeons, on the other hand, who believe that the cause of all back pain is a structural abnormality in your spine. They regard your spine as a stack of building blocks that are out of alignment. Just as it is unrealistic to think that the cause of all back pain is in your mind, however, it is unrealistic to think that the cause of all back pain is structural. It is certainly more logical that these factors work together in causing your back pain, and that in turn, the treatment of both is very important to improve your pain and your life. Looking at just one or the other is like looking at a Picasso painting with one eye closed.

Spine surgeons are notorious for ignoring the connection of psychology and back pain. The training to become a spine surgeon is rigorous and time-consuming. It requires tremendous and detailed knowledge of anatomy, as well as an enormous amount of information about surgery and ever-changing technology. In many cases, spine surgeons simply do not have enough time to be trained in psychology and its possible pain-related effects on the spine. Most spine surgeons will instead rely on a psychologist to evaluate and treat their patients when it comes to anxiety and depression. In fact, many spine surgeons will avoid treating a patient who exhibits an obvious and severe psychological condition.

PAIN AND ITS PSYCHOLOGICAL EFFECTS

Pain is a very complex process that can lead to multiple undesired effects on your body. The word pain comes from the Latin word "poena," which means penalty. This penalty is similar to an alarm that is set off by your body to inform you of the damaging effect of a process. On an evolutionary basis, pain is an extremely important tool for protection. If pain were not present, you would be bruised and often bleeding.

The significance of pain can be well illustrated by a disease called *congenital insensitivity to pain* (CIP), in which the person does not feel any pain. People with CIP usually don't survive past the age of twenty-five, since they suffer from multiple injuries. They can bite off their own fingers without any pain or discomfort. This disease points to the protective quality of pain in our lives. Unfortunately, however, excessive exposure to pain can cause immediate effects such as nausea, headaches, dizziness, weakness, drowsiness, abdominal discomfort, and perspiration, among many others. Pain can cause you to feel anger, depression, mood swings, or irritability. Severe pain can even cause you to have suicidal ideations.

Our understanding of pain, in general, is only in its infancy. Scientific research is focused on understanding pain at its cellular and molecular level. Our knowledge of how pain is perceived by the brain is incomplete. But such knowledge is important, since it can explain how the somatic perception of pain is wired in our brains. Once we understand this relationship, we will have a better idea how pain is compounded by emotional or psychological factors.

Acute Pain

Acute pain results from any disease or process that causes pain for up to three months. Acute pain is self-limiting and has an end point when the damaging injury heals or the disease resolves. Acute pain, as opposed to chronic pain, will have an identifiable cause such as surgery, traumatic injury (fracture or ligament tear), or transient headaches. If you suffer from a sprained ankle, for example, it will cause acute pain. In most cases, your pain will substantially improve after six weeks and the acute pain will resolve without the long-term effects of chronic pain. The healing of the sprain represents an end point to your acute pain.

Chronic Pain

Chronic pain is defined as pain that persists past three months and is regarded by some doctors as a disease in itself. Chronic pain usually occurs with conditions that persist for a long time. Sometimes it continues after the injury has resolved or healed. Your nervous system reacts to the memory of the initial disease or injury and continues to trigger a pain response even though the injury may not still be present. Chronic pain is a complex and poorly understood process, although some experts suggest that certain people are predisposed to chronic pain based on their gender, ethnicity, and genetics. See the boxed inset titled "The Role of Race," above, for an example of this theory.

It can be difficult to figure out the fundamental cause of chronic pain. In some cases, the honest answer from your doctor may be that she does not know where the pain is coming from. Be wary of doctors who "manufacture" a theory to explain the cause of your pain. If your doctor offers explanations that don't make sense, it should set off alarms in your mind.

Your pain may begin to dictate your daily activities and your social life. This causes further isolation and sensitization to pain. You should

The Role of Race

Another factor, when it comes to the experience of pain, is racial background. Studies have shown that there may be racial differences in the experience of pain intensity. Generally, some pain management specialists have suggested that African-Americans feel more pain as compared to Caucasians, though newer studies have challenged that. By contrast, Asians are thought to feel comparatively less intense pain with similar procedures. Overall, the sensation of pain is complex, multifactorial, and poorly understood.

attempt to avoid this isolation, since it can cause an exaggerated response to your pain. Avoidance behavior and changes to your lifestyle open the door to the transition from acute to chronic pain.

The Brain's Relationship to Pain

Frustration results from the constant experience of pain and the inability to control it. Your brain will release chemicals to combat the pain naturally, but many times this constant exposure to pain with frustration results in depression, which itself can be a symptom of chronic pain.

Animal studies have been very conclusive in showing that depression and behavioral changes may develop from frustration and constant subjection to pain that does not resolve. This frustration leads to changes in your behavior, goals, relationships, and worsening of your mental health. In fact, frustration can lead to structural changes in your brain that can actually be detected by repeated MRI studies. This demonstrates that emotions and pain can actually manifest as physical changes in your body.

If the circuitry of your brain actually changes, your brain can get sensitized to stimulation that would not otherwise have caused pain. Minor pain that is perceived as severe can produce the same effects as a severe injury. This can result in the psychological phenomenon of misunderstood pain. People around you can be very understanding of your pain if it resulted from a tangible injury such as a fracture or a recent surgery. Most people, including some of your doctors, however, will not be very accommodating to complaints of pain that are not the direct effect of an injury. Can that result in depression and frustration? It certainly can! You may be suffering from both the frustration of unexplained pain, in addition to a "support" group that is skeptical about your pain.

Your emotions are tightly connected to the sensory sections of your brain. Avoiding activities you would normally enjoy causes further emotional insult, which leads to more depression, sensitization to pain, and a lower threshold of pain. This is the model for exaggerated pain perception that has been described by some books and doctors. If you avoid activities in your daily routine because of pain, your body can get even more deconditioned, which will in turn cause more inactivity, isolation, and depression. And if you were injured at work, the injury may not allow you to return to work. Or, for legal reasons, your employer may not allow you to return to your previous job. This can cause further inactivity, isolation, and escalation of your pain.

Because of this model, most doctors will not suggest inactivity and rest. I always encourage my patients to get involved in the community, at work, or on an important project. Activities that take your mind away from your pain will keep you from constantly concentrating on your back condition. You should consider pursuing hobbies, and getting involved with projects that offer moderate physical activity and that allow you to be flexible with how much time you devote to them. This will get your mind away from your pain and help in conditioning your body. If at all possible, attempt to work, remain functional, and stay involved!

DEPRESSION AND PAIN —
A VICIOUS CYCLE

Which comes first, the chicken or the egg? This is similar to the question of which comes first, depression or pain. There is evidence to support both theories. Depression, however, is not synonymous with pain. That is, if you have pain, you are not necessarily a victim of depression. You can easily imagine, however, that you could feel depressed if you were constantly subjected to pain. If you have chronic pain, you are four times more likely to develop depression than a person who is not experiencing the sensation of pain.

The diagnosis of depression can be a difficult task in itself. You and your doctor may not even recognize that you have depression. In fact, half of people with depression are not diagnosed with it early on in its development. If you are like most other people who have depression, your initial complaint may be another illness altogether, such as pelvic pain, fibromyalgia, headache, irritable bowel syndrome, or chronic fatigue syndrome. Unfortunately, most doctors will begin by looking at physical explanations of your complaints, as opposed to depression. When the treatment for depression is effective, however, your pain and your physical complaints may improve as well. It is a known fact that the severity of your physical complaints is directly related to the severity of your depression. The worse your depression, the more pain you will experience and the more your physical complaints are likely to bother you. To you, the pain is real, but your doctors may not understand this phenomenon.

Depression can wear you down and allow you to regress into a world of loneliness and seclusion. If you have this condition, your sleep pattern is most likely affected as well. Oversleeping or not sleeping at all are signs of depression and anxiety. Overeating or loss of appetite are also common manifestations of depression and anxiety. Other symptoms include fatigue, lack of sexual interest, avoidance of relationships, or general lack of motivation. Depression will deprive you of enjoying the activities that usually result in much joy in your life. This results in avoidance of your daily routine. For instance, if you have always enjoyed reading the newspaper in the morning, you will find yourself not doing that any longer. Moreover, depression can be destructive to your personal relationships. Your spouse may not want to be around you and you may find yourself ambivalent about the distant relationship.

Pain can cause similar changes in your life. Unfortunately, back pain can mask the effects of depression. The people around you may not understand the changes in your behavior resulting from depression. It is much easier for a depressed person to explain the changes in her behavior based on back pain. A diagnosed structural abnormality in your back will justify pain and explain behavioral changes that are in fact symptomatic of depression. Unfortunately, you may not even recognize this yourself. The processes in your brain are very complex and depression may cause pain that is indistinguishable from back pain. Your psychological injury can feed the structural injury and vice versa. This vicious cycle can be detrimental to you, your family, and your career.

In most, but not all, cases, then, back pain results from structural and anatomical abnormality, which is then worsened by psychological factors. To resolve your back pain, you must treat the structural abnormality in your spine, along with any psychological issues that may be worsening your situation. It is possible that a structural abnormality such as a small herniated disc or minor arthritis will not cause you to have any pain. There are many people who have multiple small disc herniations and don't even know it. The fact is that not all spinal abnormalities result in pain. A psychological stressor, however, can cause minor pain to turn major. Resolving the psychological factor may allow you to better deal with the structural abnormality in your spine.

What makes people who have painless structural abnormalities different from other people who have agonizing pain from a small disc herniation in the lower back? Several factors can explain this. One is the person's physique and general physical condition. If you are athletic and physically well conditioned, your body is able to cope with minor abnormalities more efficiently without the sensation of pain. Another factor is your tolerance of pain and the way your brain perceives and processes pain signals. Psychological stressors can lower your pain threshold and make you more aware of minor tweaks in your back.

Depression and Surgery

It is a known fact that if you have a psychological condition such as depression or anxiety, the chances of your developing physical problems are much higher. These conditions make you more receptive to physical complaints and minor pain can become significant quite easily. For that reason, many surgeons will be reluctant to operate on you if you have a psychological condition such as depression or anxiety. When you find a surgeon who is willing to operate on you, your psychological condition reduces your chances for a successful outcome of surgery. It is well known that depression leads to lower success in patients undergoing surgery. Spinal fusion for example, is one type of surgery that most surgeons would avoid if you are severely depressed. Unfortunately, conditions that require a spinal fusion surgery are inherently painful and can cause depression. This can create a vicious cycle of pain that causes depression, which in turn can amplify pain. One process in your body feeds the other and can lead to worsening of both conditions..

The consequences of unsuccessful surgery can be devastating to both you and your surgeon. You should both do everything possible to increase your chances of success. Depression and anxiety are factors that you should attempt to resolve *before* your surgery. In fact, if you resolve these conditions, there is even a chance that you can tolerate your pain and avoid surgery altogether.

Treating the Physical Ailment and the Psychological One

Most doctors will treat you not only on the basis of your diagnosis, but also on the basis of your level of pain and discomfort. This is especially true when it comes to disorders of the spine. Diagnostic studies such as the MRI only guide your spine surgeon. The severity of your pain and your description of the changes in your life will be the determining factor in choosing the appropriate treatment modality that matches your problem. Two people may have an identical problem but exhibit very different levels of pain and dysfunction. A spine surgeon will treat them differently, since their symptoms are dissimilar.

If your surgeon is unaware of your psychological state, the risk of misdiagnosis and inappropriate treatment increases. The treatment of your psychological condition is distinct from the treatment of the structural abnormalities in your spine, but the two treatments must proceed hand in hand. Your doctor should understand your psychological condition. Most experienced doctors will attempt to treat both of these conditions.

In order to understand the treatment of depression and back pain, you must understand that the phenomenon of depression and the process of pain perception take place in your brain, which is made up of many nerves that communicate with each other constantly. The signals between the nerves are transmitted by many different chemicals. Two important chemicals in your brain are *norepinephrine* and *serotonin*. The regulation of these chemicals can improve depression, anxiety, somatization disorder, and other psychological problems. It is probably not a coincidence that the chemicals related to depression also regulate the sensation of pain in your brain. This is why pain and depression often go hand in hand. Medications that regulate these chemicals in your brain can therefore be effective in treating both pain and depression. At this time, however, no substantial differences have been established in the effectiveness of one drug over another. The chance that you will respond positively to these medications is as high as 70 percent. However, sometimes you have to try a number of different medications before you find one that works for you. If you suffer from chronic pain or depression, it is very important to get appropriate treatment for it.

You may feel that you suffer from a personal weakness if you were prescribed antidepressant medications by your doctor. You may even resist taking these medications, which can be a serious mistake. Your cultural background can play a very important role in such beliefs. Some cultures regard you as "crazy" if you use medications to control and modify your mood. In order to combat these thoughts, many people take these medications intermittently, which can be an even worse mistake.

As compared with pain medications, which most doctors would tell you to take sparingly, antidepressant medications must be taken regularly. Some of these medications will take a few weeks to begin to take effect. Many of the side effects will be worse for the first week, but will disappear as your body gets used to the medication and stabilizes. If you can tolerate the side effects, attempt to continue taking the prescribed medication until you see your doctor on the next visit. Avoid taking the medication on an intermittent basis or suddenly changing your dosage. Doing so will not raise the concentration of the medication to the expected levels in your body and can delay the desired effect.

Moreover, if you abruptly stop some of these medications, your body can react with a vengeance. Once your body gets used to an antidepressant medication, you will have to continue taking it routinely until your doctor directs you to slowly decrease its use. If you decrease the concentration of some of the medications suddenly, your depression can come back even worse than when it started. It is important to start slowly and finish slowly with these medications. You will give your brain a chance to slowly adapt to the presence or absence of the medication.

Psychotherapy and behavioral modification can supplement antidepressant medications. Alone, or in combination, psychotherapy is an effective and important part of your successful recovery. Some doctors believe that the combination of psychotherapy and medication is more successful than either one alone. Some psychologists will suggest biofeedback, hypnosis, and other relaxation techniques. Another strategy for decreasing pain and combating depression is to keep a pain diary. This diary may provide you with insight into factors that worsen your pain or depression. Educate yourself about pain and depression and think about this problem as an illness similar to other medical conditions. Get involved in your community and in your work. Avoid regression. Finally, with the blessing of your doctor, start a gradually strenuous exercise program like Pilates, yoga, or aerobics.

Somatization Disorder

You may have been diagnosed with *somatization disorder* if your doctor could not explain the reason for your physical pain based on a structural or physical condition. Your body may be expressing your emotional illness as pain in your back. To you, however, the pain is as real as if you had a structural abnormality in your spine. Your risk of having this problem is higher if this condition runs in your family. If you are a woman with a family history of this disorder, you are even more likely to have it. If you are a man with a family history of this condition, you are more likely to develop alcoholism and depression.

This condition is a chronic one. Somatization disorder usually starts in your late twenties or early thirties. The problem can last for many years and diagnosis can be difficult. You may have been subjected to extensive medical testing in the search for the cause of your pain. If you have been diagnosed with somatization disorder, you are still not immune to other physical ailments, however. Other illnesses can create confusion, since most physicians are likely to blame all of your concerns on somatization disorder. One of the symptoms of this disorder is back pain. Other symptoms of somatization disorder can include headaches, stomachache, erectile dysfunction, paralysis, weakness, and even seizures.

Once you have been diagnosed with this disorder, the treatment is focused on the secondary problems, such as abnormal social functioning, problems at work, or issues with your personal relationships. Psychotherapy and medications are medical interventions that can control your symptoms and increase your level of functioning. You will probably find psychotherapy very slow in producing results. You must realize, however, that your complaints have been present for many years and psychotherapy will take some time in unraveling them. Antidepressant medications can reduce your symptoms but are unlikely to resolve this chronic condition completely.

*   *   *

In conclusion, if you are suffering from pain and depression, rest assured that you are not alone. It's a widespread public health problem. Of all the patients who go to the office of a family practice doctor, 46 percent have a psychiatric ailment. Fortunately, you have a good chance of improving your life with the available treatment options.

Conclusion

They are all around you—people who already had spine surgery and were successful in improving their lives, their relationships, and their finances. These people no longer talk about their success. They have actually forgotten about the fact that they had surgery and got rid of their pain and dysfunction. Their victories are silent ones.

On the other hand, it is a well-known fact that surgical risks exist with any type of procedure. As we've discussed in this book, the risks for spine surgery are higher than for other types of procedures. Patients whose procedures had unfortunate outcomes remain the most vocal portion of the people who have undergone spine surgery. Don't judge the outcome of spine surgery by listening to one or two people who had bad outcomes. Talk to your doctors or ask to speak to some patients who have gone through the same procedure.

Rest assured that the outcome of most surgical procedures on the spine is favorable and the majority of patients express gratitude to their spine surgeons. Studies indicate that most patients say they would undergo the surgery again if they were placed in the same situation as before the procedure.

If you picked up this book in preparation for your surgery, I trust you have found answers to most of your questions. As your knowledge grows, you will undoubtedly have even more informed questions for your spine surgeon. You must analyze the risks, the benefits, and the alternatives to the treatment that was suggested by your surgeon. Remember, even your surgeon may not be able to answer all of your questions. Many patients ask me if I think that they should have the surgery. In most cases, I inform my patients that they are the only person who can gauge their level of pain and dysfunction. Your surgeon does not have the limitations with which you are coping. Ultimately, *you* have to make the decision if you should or should not proceed with the surgery, based on the information that you have gathered.

Some general guidelines apply, however, in most cases. If you can tolerate the pain or dysfunction, and if you can control the symptoms conservatively, you should avoid surgery. If you do not improve after a few months, you are unlikely to improve with time. That's when you should start looking into surgical options.

Many patients decide to proceed with surgery out of fear that their pain will worsen as they age. A number of patients who come to my office are terrified, for example, by the fear of becoming paralyzed by a herniated disc. Although possible, this scenario is very uncommon. Disc herniations tend to improve over time and not worsen. Preventative spine surgery is extremely rare. No spine doctor can predict the future. Some conditions like adolescent scoliosis may require surgery to prevent worsening, but this applies only to a few specific conditions that are far less common than herniated discs, arthritis, or spondylolisthesis.

You should consider the risks versus the benefits of the surgery, but keep in mind that not all of the benefits may be obvious to you before having the surgery. If you are suffering from a spinal condition that causes constant pain or the inability to walk or perform your daily activities, you are at an obvious risk of developing psychological problems. The development of anxiety and depression can be detrimental to your well-being. Constant and prolonged exposure to pain can lead to long-term consequences that may not resolve even after successful surgery. For that reason, you should consider all of the information you gathered in your decision-making process.

Feel comfortable with getting a second opinion. If your spine surgeon is competent and confident, he will welcome a second opinion. Don't worry about hurting the feelings of your doctor and concentrate on your goal of achieving a pain-free life that is joyful.

If you come to the decision to proceed with surgery, learn as much as you can about your specific surgery. Your surgeon will be happy to know that you have taken an active role in understanding your ailment and the treatment for it. It is a known fact that patients who are better informed have better outcomes. Your motivation level will improve and your anxiety about the eventual outcome will decrease. Your expectations will be more realistic and you can plan your future more effectively.

As the technology of spinal surgery evolves, new ideas are introduced. Not all have been proven to be effective and not all result in favorable outcomes. Make sure that your surgeon is knowledgeable about new technology and, if possible, avoid completely new treatment options. In some cases, new technology has later been found to be flawed, resulting in catastrophic outcomes for many people. It usually takes a year or two to understand the outcome of new technology. If a procedure or implant is successful, good reviews will be provided by that time and the technology will be in widespread use.

Many patients ask me how long it will take to recover from surgery. In turn, I ask them to define the term recovery. Understanding the details and the possible outcomes of a procedure can lead to different definitions. Take, for example, a microdiscectomy procedure. Most people will walk right after surgery. Does recovery mean walking, or does it mean becoming completely pain-free? In my opinion, neither is an accurate assessment of recovery. In most cases, recovery means reaching a plateau in improvement after surgery. Knowledge about the procedure can illuminate this, since recovery may have a different meaning for every person.

In summary, stay focused, knowledgeable, and informed. The odds are working in your favor that you will have a successful outcome with or without surgery. I thank you for taking the time to understand some of the very complex issues in the field of spine surgery, and I hope that the book has brought you many steps closer to success.

Selected References

An, Howard S. *Synopsis of Spine Surgery*. Baltimore: Williams & Wilkins, 1998.

An, Howard S. and Jenis, Louis G. *Complications of Spine Surgery: Treatment and Prevention*. Philadelphia: Lippincott Williams & Wilkins, 2006.

Buttermann, G.R. "Treatment of Lumbar Disc Herniation: Epidural Steroid Injection Compared with Discectomy: A Prospective, Randomized Study." *Journal of Bone and Joint Surgery (American)* 86(2004): 670–679.

Cheh, G., Bridwell, K.H., Lenke, L.G., Buchowski, J.M., Daubs, M.D., Kim, Y., and Baldus, C. "Adjacent Segment Disease Following Lumbar/Thoracolumbar Fusion with Pedicle Screw Instrumentation: A Minimum 5-year Follow-up." *Spine* 32(20)(2007): 2253–2257.

Clark, Charles R. *The Cervical Spine*, Fourth edition. Philadelphia: Lippincott Williams & Wilkins, 2005.

Fardon, David F. and Garfin, Steven R. *Orthopaedic Knowledge Update: Spine 2*. Rosemont, Ill.: American Academy of Orthopaedic Surgeons, 2002.

Fountas, K.N., Kapsalaki, E.Z., Nikolakakos, L.G., Smisson, H.F., Johnston, K.W., Grigorian, A.A., Lee, G.P., and Robinson, J.S. Jr. "Anterior Cervical Discectomy and Fusion Associated Complications." *Spine* 32(21)(2007): 2310–2317.

Frymoyer, John W., Ducker, Thomas B., Hadler, Nortin M., Kostuik, John P., Weinstein, James N., and Whitecloud, Thomas S. III. *The Adult Spine: Principles and Practice*, Second edition. Philadelphia: Lippincott Williams & Wilkins, 1997.

Herkowitz, H.N., and Kurz, L.T. "Degenerative Lumbar Spondylolisthesis with Spinal Stenosis: A Prospective Study Comparing Decompression with Decompression and Intertransverse Process Arthrodesis." *Journal of Bone and Joint Surgery (American)* 73(1991): 802–808.

Khalil, Tarek M., Abdel-Moty, Elsayed M., Rosomoff, Renee S., and Rosomoff, Hubert L. *Ergonomics in Back Pain: A Guide to Prevention and Rehabilitation*. Hoboken, N.J.: Wiley, 1993.

McGeary, D.D., Mayer, T.G., and Gatchel, R.J. "High Pain Ratings Predict Treatment Failure in Chronic Occupational Musculoskeletal Disorders." *Journal of Bone and Joint Surgery (American)* 88(2006): 317–325.

McLain, R.F., and Buttermann, G.R. "Epidural Steroid Injection Compared with Discectomy for the Treatment of Lumbar Disc Herniation." *Journal of Bone and Joint Surgery (American)* 87(2005): 458–459.

Meyer, T., Cooper, J., and Raspe, H. "Disabling Low Back Pain and Depressive Symptoms in the Community-Dwelling Elderly: A Prospective Study." *Spine* 32(21)(2007): 2380–2386.

Phalen, G.S., and Dickson, J.A. "Spondylolisthesis and Tight Hamstrings." *Journal of Bone and Joint Surgery (American)* 43(1961): 505–512.

Richardson, W.J., and Roush, T.F. "Internet Resources for Spine Care." *Journal of the American Academy of Orthopaedic Surgeons* 12(2004): 204.

Sarno, John E. *Healing Back Pain: The Mind-Body Connection.* New York: Warner Books, Inc., 1991.

Sever, J.W. "Disability Following Injuries to the Back in Industrial Accidents." *Journal of Bone and Joint Surgery (American)* 1(1919): 657–666.

Sobel, Dava and Klein, Arthur C. *Backache: What Exercises Work.* New York: St. Martin's Griffin, 1996.

Spivak, J.M. "Current Concepts Review—Degenerative Lumbar Spinal Stenosis." *Journal of Bone and Joint Surgery (American)* 80(1998): 1053–066.

Spivak, J.M. *Orthopaedic Knowledge Update: Spine 3.* Rosemont, Ill.: American Academy of Orthopaedic Surgeons, 2006.

Thiel, H.W., Bolton, J.E., Docherty, S., and Portlock, J.C. "Safety of Chiropractic Manipulation of the Cervical Spine: A Prospective National Survey." *Spine* 32(21)(2007): 2375–2378.

Tropiano, P., Huang, R.C., Girardi, F.P., Cammisa, F.P. Jr., and Marnay, T. "Lumbar Total Disc Replacement." *Journal of Bone and Joint Surgery (American)* 88(2006): 50–64.

Vaccaro, A.R., and Garfin, S.R. "Pedicle-Screw Fixation in the Lumbar Spine." *Journal of the American Academy of Orthopaedic Surgeons* 3(1995): 263–274.

Wiltse, L.L. "The Etiology of Spondylolisthesis." *Journal of Bone and Joint Surgery (American)* 44(1962): 539–560.

Resource List

A variety of websites can provide a broad range of resources for your health. Many of these sites relate specifically to concerns about back problems and treatment. Each of the following sites offers unique and specific information and services that may prove useful to you. You may wish to visit some of them as you determine your course of back treatment and whether back surgery is right for you.

American Academy of Orthopaedic Surgeons

Website: www.aaos.org

The official site of the American Academy of Orthopaedic Surgeons serves as a useful resource for orthopedic surgeons, who can search for articles and thus broaden their medical education. In addition, patients can search for orthopedic surgeons in their area.

American Board of Orthopaedic Surgery

Website: www.abos.org

The American Board of Orthopaedic Surgery certifies orthopedic surgeons, and its official site can provide information about your doctor's board certification.

e-Spinedoctor.com

Website: www.espinedoctor.com

The official site of Edwin Haronian, MD, discusses common disorders and treatments and provides information about operative and non-operative treatment options with useful schematics and pictures. It also provides information about the practice of Edwin Haronian, MD, and other useful information.

Google Scholar

Website: www.scholar.google.com

Recently introduced by Google, this site is a search engine for scientific information.

MD Nationwide

Website: www.mdnationwide.org

For a fee, this site provides information about doctors, including their malpractice track records.

MedlinePlus

Website: www.nlm.nih.gov/medlineplus

This site is a comprehensive and trusted source of information about all aspects of health care, including back pain.

Medscape

Website: www.medscape.com

Featuring scientific articles and references related to all aspects of health care, this is a very useful site for physicians and patients.

North American Spine Society

Website: www.spine.org

The official site of the North American Spine Society is a respected resource for both physicians and patients.

Spine Universe

Website: www.spineuniverse.com

Physicians can pay to be marketed on this commercial site, which provides free information to patients. Most of the information is reliable and accurate but can be tinged by the effects of marketing.

Web MD

Website: www.webmd.com

This site is a resource for general information about your health.

Index

Abnormal micromotion, 26
Academic hospitals, 97–98
ACDF. *See* Anterior cervical discectomy and fusion (ACDF).
Acceleration injury. *See* Whiplash.
Acetaminophen, 117
Aches, postsurgical. *See* Pain, postsurgical.
Acidosis, 144
Acupressure, 44, 46
Acupuncture, 46
Acute infection. *See* Infection, acute.
Acute pain, psychological effects of, 152
Addiction
    to exercise, 144–145
    to pain medication, 41
ADR surgery. *See* Lumbar artificial disc replacement (ADR) surgery.
Advance directives, prior to surgery, 104–105
Advil, 38
AIDS, and risk of surgical infection, 57
ALIF. *See* Anterior lumbar interbody fusion (ALIF).
Allo-grafting, 63
Ambien, 42
Ambulation training, 127
Ambulatory surgery center. *See* Outpatient or ambulatory surgery center (ASC).
American Academy of Orthopaedic Surgeons, 95, 141
American Board of Medical Specialties, 92
American Board of Neurological Surgery, 92
American Board of Orthopaedic Surgery, 92

American College of Sports Medicine, 141
American Red Cross, 108
Amitriptyline. *See* Elavil.
Anatomy of back, 7–17
    discs, 14
    ligaments, 15–16
    muscles, 17
    neural foramen, 15
    sections of spine, 8–12
    spinal cord, 8
    vertebrae, 12–13
Andrews table, 71, 116
Anesthesia, 111–113
    complications, 61
    general, 111–112
    local, 116–117
    regional, 112–113
    skin, 113
    spinal, 112–113
Annulus, 14, 20, 52
Ansaid, 38
Anterior cervical discectomy and fusion (ACDF), 64–66
Anterior longitudinal ligament, 15–16
Anterior lumbar interbody fusion (ALIF), 77–78
Anti-inflammatory drugs
    side effects, 39–40
    varieties, 38
Aquatherapy, 45
Arthritis
    defined, 19–20
    degenerative, 9
    and scoliosis, 35
    and spondylolysis, 27
    and stenosis, 26

Arthropathy. *See* Facet hypertrophy.
Arthrotec, 38
Artificial disc, 83
ASC. *See* Outpatient or ambulatory
    surgery center (ASC).
Aspirin, 39
Asthma, 100
Atlanto-axial rotation, 10
Atlas (C1), 8, 10
Auto-grafting, 63
Autologous blood transfusion, 107–108
Axis (C2), 8, 10

Back
    anatomy of, 7–17
    function of, 18
Back problems, determining causes of,
    19–35
    arthritis, 19–20
    cancer, 33
    deformity, 34–35
    disc herniation, 11, 20–25
    infection, 33–34
    spinal stenosis, 26
    spondylolisthesis, 27–29
    spondylolysis, 27–28
    traumatic injuries, 29–32
Bacteria-fighting mechanisms, natural, 122
Benefits of exercise. *See* Exercise,
    benefits of.
Bengay, 43
Black disc, 20
Bleeding, gastric, 39
Blood, volunteer-donated, 108
Blood cells, 106–107
Blood clot, 61
Blood donation, preoperative. *See*
    Autologous blood transfusion.
Blood patch, 58
Blood transfusions, 106–110
    autologous blood transfusion, 107–108
    Cell Saver, 109
    directed blood donation, 109
    hemodilution, 109–110
    volunteer-donated blood, 108
BMP. *See* Bone morphogenetic protein
    (BMP), 63
Board certification of your surgeon, 92
Bone, cancellous, 79
Bone grafting, 63

Bone morphogenetic protein (BMP), 63
Bone scan, 34
Brace. *See* Lumbar corset.
Brain's relationship to pain, 153–154
Burst fracture. *See* Fracture, burst.

C1. *See* Atlas (C1).
C2. *See* Axis (C2).
Calcium, 146
Cancellous bone, 79
Cancer, as cause of back problems, 33
Capsin, 43
Cardiac stress test, 99
Cauda equina, 12
Cauda equina syndrome, 12, 70
CBC. *See* Complete blood count (CBC).
Celebrex, 39
Celestone, 48
Cell Saver, 109
Cement, surgical, 124
Central nervous system, 7
Cerebral palsy, 34
Cerebrospinal fluid, 8, 57–58
Certification of your surgeon, 92
Cervical disc
    herniation, 22–23
    replacement, 69
Cervical fracture, 29
Cervical laminectomy, 67–68
Cervical laminoplasty, 68
Cervical lordosis, 8, 9
Cervical myelopathy, 64
Cervical spine (neck), 8–9, 10–11
Cervical spine surgeries, 64–69
    anterior cervical discectomy and
        fusion (ACDF), 64–66
    cervical disc replacement, 69
    cervical laminectomy, 67–68
    posterior cervical foraminotomy, 66–67
    posterior cervical fusion, 68–69
Cervical sprain syndrome. *See* Whiplash.
Cervical stenosis, 26–27
Charité artificial disc, 83
Chest, importance of, to posture, 133
Chiropractic manipulation, 45–46
Choices regarding surgeon and care
        facility, 89–98
    facility, 95–98
    surgeon, 90–95
Cholesterol, 143, 146

Chronic infection. *See* Infection, chronic.
Chronic pain, psychological effects of, 152–154
Circumferential fusion, 76
Clearance. *See* Preoperative medical clearance.
Clinoril, 38
Clot, blood, 61
CNS. *See* Central nervous system.
Coccyx. *See* Sacrum/coccyx.
Codeine, 41, 117
Cold laser, 44
Cold therapy, 44
Complete blood count (CBC), 107
Complications, postsurgical, 119–125
    deep venous thrombosis (DVT), 124–125
    fever, 120–121
    pulmonary embolism (PE), 124–125
    swelling, 120
    wound infections, 121–124
Complications, surgical, 61
Compression fracture. *See* Fracture, compression.
Computed Tomography scan. *See* CT scan.
Conservative treatment. *See* Nonsurgical treatment options.
Consultation, making the most of, 24
Conus medullaris, 12
Core exercises, 47
Corset. *See* Lumbar corset.
Cortical bone, 79
Cortisone, 40, 48, 49, 60, 101
Cox-2 inhibitors, 39
CSF. *See* Cerebrospinal fluid.
CT scan, 15
CT-discogram, 52
CT-myelogram, 22
Cycle of depression and pain, 154–160
    relationship to surgery, 156–157
    somatization disorder, 159–160
    treating both physical and psychological ailments, 157–159
Cyst, synovial, 61

Dalmane, 42
Daypro, 38
Decompression surgery, 61–62
Decortication, 79
Deep breathing, 104
Deep venous thrombosis (DVT), 124–125

Deformity
    kyphosis, 35
    scoliosis, 34–35
Degenerative arthritis. *See* Arthritis, degenerative.
Degenerative disc disease, 20
Demerol, 118
Dens, 10
Dependency on pain medication, 41
Depo-Medrol, 40, 48
Depression, 143–144, 154–160
DePuy Spine Inc., 83
Dexamethasone, 40
Diabetes, 33, 57, 61, 100, 143
Diet, in preparation for surgery, 101–102
Directed blood donation, 109
Disc, artificial, 83
Disc, black, 20
Disc, vertebral, 7, 14
    bulge of, 21
    extrusion of, 21
    herniation of, 11, 20–25
    protrusion of, 21
Disc disease, degenerative, 20
Discectomy, 61
    endoscopic, 75
    microendoscopic, 61, 73–74
    percutaneous, 74–75
Discitis, 15, 33–34, 64
Discogenic pain, 14
Discogram, 51–52, 57
Dislocation, 32
Doctor. *See* Surgeon, choosing.
Driving, and posture, 137–138
Drugs. *See* Medications.
Dura, 8
Durable power of attorney. *See* Power of attorney, durable.
Duragesic patch, 43
Dural tear, 57–58
DVT. *See* Deep venous thrombosis (DVT).

Echocardiogram, 99
EKG. *See* Electrocardiogram (EKG).
Elavil, 42
Electrocardiogram (EKG), 98
Electromyography (EMG), 22
Endorphins, 144
Endoscopic discectomy. *See* Discectomy, endoscopic.

Endurance training, 142
Epidural
    anesthesia, 113
    catheter, 117
    injection, 48–49, 57
Erector spinae, 17
Ergonomics
    chair, 135–136
    workstation, 137
Exercise, benefits of, 142–145
    "addiction" to, 144–145
    bones and muscles, 142
    cholesterol and diabetes, 143
    depression, 143–144
    libido, 143
Exercise guidelines, 141–142
Exercises, core, 47
Existing health problems, 99–100
Extremity pain, 21
Extruded disc. *See* Disc extrusion.

Facet arthropathy. *See* Facet hypertrophy.
Facet block, 49–50
Facet hypertrophy, 13
Facet joint, 11
Facet syndrome. *See* Facet hypertrophy.
Facetectomy, medial, 70
Facility, choosing, 95–98
    academic hospitals, 97–98
    outpatient or ambulatory surgery
        centers (ASCs), 96–97
Feet, importance of, to posture, 132
Feldene, 38
Fellowship, of your surgeon, 90–92
Fever, postsurgical, 120–121
Flat back syndrome, 9–10
Flexibility, 18
    training for, 142
Fluoroscopy, 48, 50, 51, 53
Foley catheter, 120
Food and Drug Administration, 38, 69,
    83–84
Foramen
    neural, 14, 15
    stenosis of, 15
    transverse, 10
Foraminotomy, 61, 72
Fracture, 30–32
    burst, 32
    cervical, 29

compression, 31
    odontoid, 31
    and scoliosis, 35
Fusion surgery, 61–63
    circumferential, 76
    lumbar, 75–85
    minimally invasive, 82–83

Gabapentin. *See* Neurontin.
Gallium scan, 34
Gastric bleeding. *See* Bleeding, gastric.
Gastric ulcers. *See* Ulcers, gastric.
Gastritis, 39, 40
General anesthesia. *See* Anesthesia,
    general.
Grafting, of bone, 63
Guided relaxation. *See* Relaxation, guided.

Hamstrings, importance of, to posture,
    133–134
Harrington rod, 10
Headphones, 137
Health problems, existing, 99–100
Health-care proxy, 105
Heart attack, 61
Heat therapy, 44
Hematrocit, 107
Hemodilution, 109–110
Hemoglobin, 107
Hepatitis, 108
Herniated nucleus pulposus. *See*
    Herniation, disc.
Herniation, disc, 11, 20–25
    caused by lifting, 139–140
    cervical, 22–23
    epidural for, 48
    lumbar, 24–25
HIV
    risk from blood transfusion, 108
    and risk of spine infection, 33, 34,
    and risk of surgical infection, 57
HMO plans. *See* Insurance and HMO
    plans.
HNP. *See* Herniation, disc.
Home help, postsurgery, 126–127
Hospitals
    academic, 97–98
    specialty, 97
Humpback. *See* Kyphosis (humpback).
Hydrocodone, 117

Hygiene, in preparation for surgery, 102–103
Hyperextension injury. *See* Whiplash.
Hypertension, 100
Hypertrophy. *See* Facet hypertrophy.

Ibuprofen, 117
Ibuprofin, 38
Icy Hot, 43
IDET. *See* Intradiscal electrothermal therapy (IDET).
Iliocostalis muscle, 17
Iliolumbar ligament, 16
Incentive spirometer, 120
Indocin, 38
Infection, as a cause of back problems, 33–34
Infection, as a result of back surgery, 56–57
  acute, 124
  chronic, 124
Injectable pain medications, 118
Injuries, traumatic, 29–32
  dislocations, 32
  fractures, 30–32
  sprains, strains, and whiplash, 29–30
Inpatient procedures, 106
Insurance and HMO plans, 94–95
Interferential muscle stimulation unit, 44
Internal disc derangement, 20
Interspinous ligament, 16
Intertransverse ligament, 16
Intradiscal electrothermal therapy (IDET), 52–54
Irrigation and debridement, 123–124

Kidney damage/failure, 39
Kyphoplasty, 62, 85–86
Kyphosis (humpback), 8, 9, 35

Lamina, 13, 27, 67–68
Laminectomy, 61
  cervical, 67–68
  lumbar, 70–71
Laminoplasty, 61
  cervical, 68
Laminotomy, 61, 72
Laparoscopic surgery, 82
Laser discectomy, 61, 74
Lateral mass, 11
Lateral mass screws, 68

Legs, importance of, to posture, 132
Libido, 143
Lidocaine, 43
Lidoderm patch, 43
Life-support machines, 105
Lifting, 139–140
Ligaments, 15–16
  injury to, 29, 30
Ligamentum flavum, 15, 16
  and stenosis, 26
Litigation, regarding your surgeon, 94
Liver damage, 39
Living will, 105
Local anesthesia. *See* Anesthesia, local.
Lodine, 38
Longissimus muscle, 17
Lordosis, 8
Low back pain, 14
Lower back. *See* Lumbar spine.
Lumbar artificial disc replacement (ADR) surgery, 83–85
Lumbar brace. *See* Lumbar corset.
Lumbar corset, 140
Lumbar decompressive procedures, 70–75
  endoscopic discectomy, 75
  laser discectomy, 74
  lumbar laminectomy, 70–71
  lumbar microdiscectomy and laminotomy, 71–73
  microendoscopic discectomy, 73–74
  minimally invasive microdiscectomy, 73–74
  nucleoplasty, 75
  percutaneous discectomy, 74–75
Lumbar disc herniation, 24
Lumbar fusion, 75–85
  anterior lumbar interbody fusion (ALIF), 77–78
  lumbar artificial disc replacement (ADR) surgery, 83–85
  minimally invasive fusions, 82–83
  posterior lumbar interbody fusion (PLIF), 80–81
  posterior lumbar fusion (PLF), 78–79
  techniques, comparison of, 82
  transforaminal lumbar interbody fusion (TLIF), 80–81
Lumbar laminectomy, 70–71
Lumbar lordosis, 8

Lumbar microdiscectomy and
    laminotomy, 71–73
Lumbar spinal stenosis, 27
Lumbar spine, 8–9, 11–12, 13, 14
Lumbar spine surgeries, 69–85
    lumbar decompressive procedures,
        70–75
    lumbar fusion, 75–85
Lumbar support corset. *See* Lumbar corset.
Lumbosacral ligament, 16
Lyrica, 42

Magnetic resonance imaging. *See* MRI.
Malpractice, 94
Marcaine, 116–117
Massage therapy, 44
"Matter alone matters," 150–151
Mattress, selecting, 138–139
Mechanical pain, 21
Medial facetectomy. *See* Facetectomy,
    medial.
Medical and anesthetic complications.
    See Complications, surgical.
Medical clearance. *See* Preoperative
    medical clearance.
Medications, 38–43
    anti-inflammatory drugs, 38–40
    muscle relaxants, 40
    nerve-stabilizing medications, 42
    oral medications, 117
    pain medications, 41–42
    sleep medications, 42
    topical medications, 43
Meditation, 104
Methylprednisolone, 40
METRx instrument system, 73–74
Microdiscectomy, 61, 62
    minimally invasive, 73–74
Microdiscectomy and laminotomy,
    lumbar, 71–73
Microendoscopic discectomy. *See*
    Discectomy, microendoscopic.
Micromotion, abnormal, 26
Midback. *See* Thoracic spine.
Midline axial pain, 21
"Mind over pain," 150
Mineralization, 146
Minimally invasive fusions. *See* Fusion
    surgery, minimally invasive.
Minimally invasive microdiscectomy.

    See Microdiscectomy, minimally
    invasive.
Mobic, 38
Morphine, 41, 118
Motrin, 38
MRI, 14
Muscle relaxants, 40
Muscle training, the three aspects of, 142
Muscles, back, 17
Music therapy, 104
Myelogram, 22
Myelopathy, 23
    cervical, 64

Naprosyn, 38
Narcotics, 41
NCV. *See* Nerve conduction velocity
    (NCV).
Neck. *See* Cervical spine (neck).
Neck pain. *See* Pain, neck.
Nerve conduction velocity (NCV), 22
Nerve-stabilizing medications, 42
Neural foramen. *See* foramen, neural.
Neurological injury, 59–60
Neurontin, 42
Noninvasive therapies, 43–47
    acupuncture, 46
    chiropractic manipulation, 45–46
    physical therapy, 44–45
    Pilates, 46–47
    yoga, 46–47
Nonmechanical pain. *See* Pain,
    nonmechanical.
Nonsteroidal anti-inflammatory drugs
    (NSAIDs), 38–40
Nonsurgical treatment options, 37–54
    medications, 38–43
    other noninvasive therapies, 43–47
    pain management procedures, 47–54
Norco, 41, 117
North American Spine Society, 95
NSAIDs. *See* Nonsteroidal anti-
    inflammatory drugs (NSAIDs).
Nucleoplasty, 75
Nucleus pulposus, 14, 20
Nutrition, 146

Odontoid fracture. *See* Fracture, odontoid.
Old theories of back pain psychology,
    persistence of, 149–151

"Matter alone matters," 150–151
"Mind over pain," 150
Opiates, 41
Opioid pain patch. See Patch, opioid
    pain.
OPLL, 27
Oral medications. See Medications, for
    treatment of back problems, oral.
Orudis, 38
Oruvail, 38
Ossification of Posterior Longitudinal
    Ligament. See OPLL.
Osteogenesis imperfecta, 34
Osteomyelitis, 33–34
Osteophyte, 9, 20
Osteoporosis, 9, 85, 142
Osteoporosis insufficiency fracture. See
    Fracture, compression.
Outpatient or ambulatory surgery
    center (ASC), 96–97
Outpatient procedures, 105–106

Pain
    acute pain, and psychological
        effects, 152
    chronic pain, and psychological
        effects, 152–154
    discogenic, 14
    extremity, 21
    low back, 14
    mechanical, 21
    midline axial, 21
    neck (cervical), 29–30
    nonmechanical, 21
    postsurgical aches and pains, 115–116
    postsurgical pain-control methods,
        116–119
    radiating, 21
Pain control methods
    epidural catheter, 117
    general medications, 41–42
    injectable pain medications, 118
    local anesthetics, 116–117
    oral medications, 117
    patient-controlled analgesia (PCA)
        pump, 118–119
Pain management procedures, 47–54
    discogram, 51–52
    epidural injection, 48–49
    facet block, 49–50

intradiscal electrothermal theraphy
    (IDET), 52–54
rhizotomy, 50–51
selective nerve root block, 49
Paralysis, 59–60
Paraplegia, 34
Patch
    blood, 58
    duragesic, 43
    opioid pain, 43
Patient-controlled analgesia (PCA)
    pump, 118–119
PE. See Pulmonary embolism (PE).
Pedicle, 13
Pedicle screw, 60, 63, 76
Pelvis, 8, 9, 12
    importance of, to posture, 133
Percocet, 41
Percutaneous discectomy. See
    Discectomy, percutaenous.
Physical therapy, 44–45
Physician. See Surgeon, choosing.
Pilates, 46–47
PLF. See Posterior lumbar fusion (PLF).
PLIF. See Posterior lumbar interbody
    fusion (PLIF).
Podiatrist, 132, 133
Posterior cervical foraminotomy, 66–67
Posterior cervical fusion, 68–69
Posterior longitudinal ligament, 16
Posterior lumbar fusion (PLF), 78–79
Posterior lumbar interbody fusion
    (PLIF), 80–81
Postsurgical recovery. See Recovery,
    postsurgical.
Postsurgical therapy. See Therapy,
    postsurgical.
Posture, improving, 131–135
    changing position often, 134–135
    chest, 133
    feet, 132
    hamstrings, 133–134
    legs, 132–133
    pelvis, 133
    shoulders, 133
Pott's disease, 34
Power of attorney, durable, 105
Pregabalin. See Lyrica.
Preoperative blood donation. See
    Autologous blood transfusion.

Preoperative medical clearance, 98–99
Preparations for surgery. *See* Surgery,
    immediate preparations for.
Preparing for surgery. *See* Surgery.
Preventing future back problems,
        131–147
    driving, 137–138
    lifting, 139–140
    nutrition, 146
    posture, improving, 131–135
    sitting, 135–137
    sleeping, 138–139
    strengthening your body, 140–145
    weight control, 146–147
Process
    spinous, 12, 13
    transverse, 13
Prodisc, 84
Pseudarthrosis, 58–59
Psychological effects of pain, 151–154
    acute, 152
    chronic, 152–154
Psychological preparation for surgery,
        103–104
Psychology and back pain, 149–160
    cycle of depression and pain, 154–160
    old theories, persistence of, 149–151
    psychological effects of pain, 151–154
Pulmonary embolism (PE), 124–125
Pulmonary function test, 99–100

Race, effect of, upon experiencing pain,
        153
Radiating pain, 21
Radical discectomy, 78
Radiculopathy, 21, 23
Recovery, postsurgical, 111–127
    anesthesia, types of, 111–113
    complications, 119–125
    home help, 126–127
    pain, 115–119
    recovery room, 114–115
    surgical wound, 119
    therapy, 127
    walking, 125–126
Recovery room, 114–115
Rectus abdominis, 141
Red blood cells, 106–107
Reflexology, 44
Regional anesthesia

    epidural anesthesia, 113
    skin anesthesia, 113
    spinal anesthesia, 112–113
Relafen, 38
Relaxants, muscle, 40
Relaxation
    guided, 104
    techniques, 104
Restoril, 42
Resuscitation, 105
Rhizotomy, 50–51
Risks of back surgery, 56–61
    dural tear, 57–58
    infection, 56–57
    medical and anesthetic
        complications, 61
    neurological injury, 59–60
    pseudarthrosis, 58–59
Robaxin, 40

Sacrum/coccyx, 8, 9
Sciatica, 25
Scoliosis, 34–35
Sections of spine. *See* Spine, sections of.
Selective nerve root block, 49
Sequential compression device, 125
Shoulders, importance of, to posture, 133
Single Photon Emission Computed
        Tomography. *See* SPECT scan.
Sitting, and posture, 135–137
    ergonomic chair, 135–136
    ergonomic workstation, 137
    headphones, 137
Skelaxin, 40
Skin anesthesia. *See* Anesthesia, skin.
Sleep medications, 42
Sleeping, and posture, 138–139
Slippage, vertebral, 28–29
Soma, 40
Somatization disorder, 159–160
Somatosensory evoked potential (SSEP).
Specialty hospitals, 97
SPECT scan, 28
Spinal anesthesia. *See* Anesthesia, spinal.
Spinal canal, 8, 10
Spinal column, 7, 8
Spinal cord, 7, 8
Spinal nerve root, 10, 14
Spinal stenosis. *See* Stenosis, spinal.
Spinalis muscle, 17

Spine, anatomy of, 7–18
Spine, sections of, 8–12
   cervical, 10–11
   lumbar, 11–12
   sacrum/coccyx, 12
   thoracic, 11
Spinous process. *See* Process, spinous.
Spirometer. *See* Incentive spirometer.
Spondylolisthesis, 27, 28–29
Spondylolysis, 27–28
Sprain, spinal, 29
SSEP. *See* Somatosensory evoked
   potential (SSEP).
Stenosis, spinal
   cervical, 26–27
   cervical laminectomy for, 67
   epidural for, 48
   lumbar, 27
Steri-Strips, 119
Steroidal anti-inflammatory
   medications, 38–40
Steroids, 101
Strain, spinal, 29
Strength training, 142
Strengthening your body, 140–145
   "addiction" to exercise, 144–145
   benefits of exercise, 142–144
   exercise guidelines, 141–142
   three aspects of muscle training, the,
     142
Stress test. *See* Cardiac stress test.
Stroke, 61
Subcuticular closure, 119
Subluxation, 32
Support corset. *See* Lumbar corset.
Supraspinous ligament, 16
Surgeon, choosing, 89–95
   board certification, 92
   insurance and HMO plans, 94–95
   litigation, 94
   practice, type of, 92–93
   training, 90–91
   websites, 95
Surgery, 89–110
   advance directives, 104–105
   blood transfusions, 106–110
   choices regarding surgeon and care
     facility, 89–98
   diet, in preparation for, 101–102
   existing health problems, 99–100

   hygiene, in preparation for, 102–103
   immediate preparations for, 99–105
   inpatient procedures, 106
   outpatient procedures, 105–106
   preoperative medical clearance, 98–99
   psychological preparation, 103–104
   steroids, 101
Surgery, types of, 61–68
   decompression surgery, 62
   fusion surgery, 63–64
   kyphoplasty, 85–86
   surgeries of the cervical spine
     (neck), 64–69
   surgeries of the lumbar spine, 69–85
   vertebroplasty, 85–86
Surgical cement. *See* Cement, surgical.
Surgical options for your back, 55–86
   risks to consider, 56–61
   types of surgery, 61–86
Surgical wound. *See* Wound, surgical.
Swelling, postsurgical, 120
Synovial cyst, 61
Synthes, 84

Tear, dural, 57–58
Theophyline, 58
Therapy
   cold, 44
   heat, 44
   massage, 44
   music, 104
   noninvasive, 43–47
   physical, 44–45
   postsurgical, 127
Thoracic kyphosis, 8, 9
Thoracic spine, 8, 9
360-degree fusion, 76
TLIF. *See* Transforaminal lumbar
   interbody fusion (TLIF).
Toelerance of pain medication, 41
Topical medications, 43
Toradol, 38
Training, muscle, 142
Training, of your surgeon, 90–91
Transforaminal lumbar interbody
   fusion (TLIF), 80–81
Transverse foramen. *See* Foramen,
   transverse.
Transverse process. *See* Process,
   transverse.

Traumatic injuries. *See* Injuries,
    traumatic.
Trocar, 85–86
Tuberculosis, 34
Tumor, 35
Tylenol #3, 117

Ulcers, gastric, 39
Ultrasound, 44
Urinary tract infection (UTI), 121

Valium, 40
Vena cava, 125
Ventilator, 111
Vertebrae, 7, 12–13
Vertebral artery, 10
Vertebral body, 12, 13, 16
Vertebroplasty, 62, 85–86
Vicodin, 41, 117
Vicoprofen, 41
Vioxx, 39
Visualization, 104

Vitamin D, 146
Voltaren, 38
Volunteer-donated blood, 108

Walking, after surgery, 125–126
Websites, 95
Weight control, 146–147
Whiplash, 15, 29–30
White blood cells, 106–107
Wilson frame, 71
Wound, surgical, 119
Wound infections, 121–124
    natural bacteria-fighting
        mechanisms, 122
    risk factors, 122–123
    signs of, 123
    treatment, 123–124

X-ray, 15

Yellow ligament. *See* Ligamentum flavum.
Yoga, 46–47

RELIEVING PAIN NATURALLY
Safe and Effective Alternative Approaches to Treating and Overcoming Chronic Pain
Sylvia Goldfarb, PhD and Roberta W. Waddell

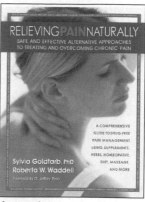

For millions of Americans, severe pain is a fact of life. Standard drug therapies may offer relief, but come with a host of side effects, and can become less effective over time. While many would prefer nondrug options, the available information on alternative treatment has long been scattered or incomplete—or it was, until now. *Relieving Pain Naturally* is a comprehensive guide to drug-free pain management. Written in nontechnical language, this up-to-date resource is designed for ease of use and quick accessibility.

Relieving Pain Naturally begins by examining thirty-seven of the most common chronic pain-related conditions, from arthritis to tendonitis. It then offers twenty-seven drug-free therapies, including both conventional and alternative treatments. A resource section guides you to professional organizations that can help you find an appropriate therapist in your area. With *Relieving Pain Naturally*, it's easy to take that first step toward side-effect-free pain relief.

$18.95 • 296 pages • 8.5 x 11-inch paperback • ISBN 978-0-7570-0079-9

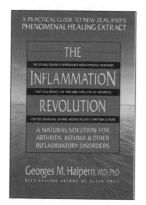

THE INFLAMMATION REVOLUTION
A Natural Solution for Arthritis, Asthma, & Other Inflammatory Disorders
Georges M. Halpern. MD, PhD

Over two decades ago, researchers observed that New Zealand's coast-dwelling Maori had a far lower incidence of arthritis-related disease than those Maori who lived inland. The cause of this was ultimately traced to the coastal Maori's consumption of green-lipped mussels. *The Inflammation Revolution* tells the story of this discovery, and presents vital information on how specific lipids found in green-lipped mussels offer benefits not only to bone joints, but to other organs as well.

With the risks of many anti-inflammatory prescription drugs continuing to make headlines, it has become vital for millions of arthritis sufferers, asthmatics, and others with inflammation-related disorders to find safer options. In *The Inflammation Revolution,* you will learn how marine lipids work, what scientific studies have shown about their use, and how this "miracle from the sea" can be used to safely relieve arthritis pain and restore better breathing to asthmatics.

$13.95 • 144 pages • 6 x 9-inch paperback • ISBN 978-0-7570-0283-0

STOPPING INFLAMMATION
Relieving the Cause of Degenerative Diseases

Nancy Appleton, PhD

Most of us think of inflammation as a symptom associated with an infection or injury. Dr. Nancy Appleton, however, has discovered that it might be more than just a simple reaction to a health disorder. When the body's tissues are disturbed in some manner, a series of complex reactions takes place, resulting in inflammation. In most cases, when the disorder stops, the tissue returns to its normal healthy state. Sometimes, though, the tissue remains chronically inflamed. Dr. Appleton's research demonstrates that this condition might be more harmful than ever suspected.

Drawing on the latest medical research, *Stopping Inflammation* begins with a full explanation of inflammation and its causes. It then looks at inflammation's role in various health disorders, from obesity to cancer. Finally, the book provides a number of nondrug treatments aimed not at controlling the problem, but at removing its cause. Here are safe and credible solutions for restoring good health.

$14.95 • 224 pages • 6 x 9-inch paperback • ISBN 978-0-7570-0148-2

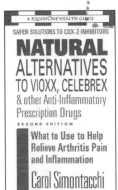

NATURAL ALTERNATIVES TO VIOXX, CELEBREX
& OTHER ANTI-INFLAMMATORY PRESCRIPTION DRUGS
What to Use to Help Relieve Arthritis Pain and Inflammation

Carol Simontacchi

Beyond today's headlines and pharmaceutical spin is an underlying truth—COX-2 inhibitor drugs can be extremely dangerous to your health. While this class of drugs does relieve pain and inflammation, the potential for heart attack and stroke has proven too great a risk for many. For those who are looking for other options, health expert Carol Simontacchi has put together a simple guide to using safer natural alternatives. Written in easy-to-understand language, this book provides solid information about nature's most effective treatments.

Clearly, there is a place for drugs, but becoming a human guinea pig should not be part of the equation. Although natural product companies may not have the advertising dollars enjoyed by the pharmaceutical industry, the beneficial effects of natural remedies should not be overlooked. *Natural Alternatives to Vioxx, Celebrex & Other Anti-Inflammatory Prescription Drugs* provides a vital resource for those looking for a safer solution.

$5.95 • 96 pages • 4 x 7-inch mass paperback • ISBN 978-0-7570-0278-6

For more information about our books,
visit our website at www.squareonepublishers.com

FOR A COPY OF OUR CATALOG, CALL TOLL FREE: 877-900-BOOK, ext. 100